Portable
Pathophysiology

Portable Pathophysiology

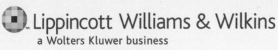
Lippincott Williams & Wilkins
a Wolters Kluwer business

Philadelphia · Baltimore · New York · London
Buenos Aires · Hong Kong · Sydney · Tokyo

STAFF

Executive Publisher
Judith A. Schilling McCann, RN, MSN

Editorial Director
H. Nancy Holmes

Clinical Director
Joan M. Robinson, RN, MSN

Senior Art Director
Arlene Putterman

Art Director
Elaine Kasmer

Editorial Project Manager
Jennifer Lynn Kowalak

Clinical Project Manager
Beverly Ann Tscheschlog, RN, BS

Editor
Julie Munden

Clinical Editors
Tamara M. Kear, RN, MSN, CNN;
Jennifer Meyering, RN, MSN, CCRN

Copy Editors
Kimberly Bilotta (supervisor),
Jane Bradford, Amy Furman,
Shana Harrington, Irene Pontarelli,
Dorothy P. Terry, Pamela Wingrod

Designers
Debra Moloshok

Digital Composition Services
Diane Paluba (manager),
Joyce Rossi Biletz, Donna S. Morris

Manufacturing
Beth J. Welsh

Editorial Assistants
Megan L. Aldinger, Karen J. Kirk,
Linda K. Ruhf

Indexer
Barbara Hodgson

Library of Congress Cataloging-in-Publication Data
Portable pathophysiology.
   p. ; cm.
  Includes bibliographical references and index.
  1. Pathology—Atlases. 2. Pathology—Handbooks, manuals, etc. I. Lippincott Williams & Wilkins. II. Title.
  [DNLM: 1. Pathology—Atlases. 2. Pathology—Handbooks. QZ 17 P839 2006]
  RB33.P67 2006
  616.07—dc22
  ISBN 1-58255-455-2 (alk. paper)   2005034581

Contents

Contributors
and consultants

Cheryl A. Bean, APRN,BC, DSN, ANP, AOCN
Associate Professor/Adult Nurse Practitioner
Indiana University School of Nursing
Indianapolis

Peggy Bozarth, RN, MSN
Professor
Hopkinsville (Ky.) Community College

Yvette P. Conley, PhD
Assistant Professor of Nursing and Human Genetics
University of Pittsburgh

Lillian Craig, RN, MSN, FNP-C
Family Nurse Practitioner
Adjunct Faculty
Oklahoma Panhandle State University
Goodwell

Shelba Durston, RN, MSN, CCRN
Nursing Instructor
San Joaquin Delta College
Stockton, Calif.
Staff Nurse
San Joaquin General Hospital
French Camp, Calif.

Ken W. Edmisson, RNC, ND, EdD, FNP
Associate Professor
Middle Tennessee State University
Murfreesboro

William F. Galvin, BA, MSEd, CRT, RRT, CPFT
Assistant Professor, School of Allied Health Professions
Program Director, Respiratory Care Program
Gwynedd Mercy College
Gwynedd Valley, Pa.

Deborah A. Hanes, RN, MSN, CNS, CRNP
Nurse Practitioner
Cleveland Clinic Foundation

JoAnne Konick-McMahan, RN, MSN, CCRN
Instructor, School of Nursing
Reading Hospital & Medical Center
West Reading, Pa.

Lt. Manuel D. Leal, PA-C (MPAS)
Department Head, Camp Smith
Hawaii
Naval Medical Clinic
Pearl Harbor, Hawaii

Dawna Martich, RN, MSN
Trainer
American Healthways
Pittsburgh

E. Ann Myers, MD, FACP, FACE
President
Golden Gate Endocrine Specialists
San Francisco

Sundaram V. Ramanan, MD,
MS, FACP, FRCP (Edinburgh)
Professor of Clinical Medicine
University of Connecticut School of
Medicine
St. Francis Hospital and Medical
Center
Hartford

Barbara L. Sauls, EdD, PA-C
Clinical Director PA Program/Faculty
King's College
Wilkes Barre, Pa.

Janet Somlyay, RN, MSN, CNS,
CPNP, Lt. Col. USAF (Ret)
Assistant Lecturer
Fay W. Whitney School of Nursing
University of Wyoming
Laramie

Sandra M. Waguespack, RN,
MSN
Instructor and Course Director
Louisiana State University Health
Sciences Center School of
Nursing
New Orleans

1

Cardiovascular system

Acute coronary syndromes

- Begins with rupture or erosion of plaque
- Results in platelet adhesions, fibrin clot formation, and activation of thrombin, which results in enlarging thrombus
- Types (as determined by degree of coronary artery occlusion): unstable angina, non–ST-segment elevation myocardial infarction (MI), or ST-segment elevation MI

Causes
- Atherosclerosis
- Embolism

Pathophysiologic changes

ANGINA

Myocardial ischemia ➡	Chest pain relieved by nitroglycerin

MI

Coronary artery occlusion ➡	Chest pain unrelieved by rest or nitroglycerin
Pain; sympathetic stimulation ➡	Perspiration, anxiety, hypertension, feeling of doom
Impaired myocardial function ➡	Fatigue, shortness of breath, cool extremities, hypotension
Pain; vagal stimulation ➡	Nausea and vomiting

CORONARY ARTERIES

Plaque — ┌ Plaque rupture

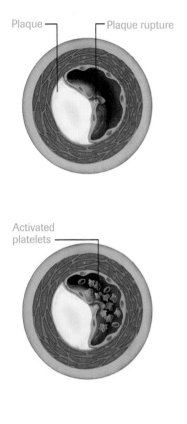

Collagen ———— ┐ ┌ ─── VW factor
Platelet ——— ┐ │ │ ┌── Thrombin

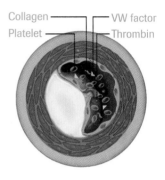

Activated
platelets ———

Thrombus ———

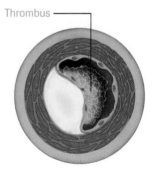

Aneurysm, abdominal aortic

- Abnormal dilation in aortic arterial wall
- Most evident as a pulsating mass in the periumbilical area
- Generally occurs between renal arteries and iliac branches
- In dissecting aneurysm, hemorrhagic separation occurring in the aortic wall; emergent situation requiring prompt surgery and stabilization
- In saccular aneurysm, results in outpouching of the arterial wall
- In fusiform aneurysm, appears as spindle-shaped and encompassing the entire aortic circumference
- In false aneurysm, occurs when the entire vessel wall is injured and leads to a sac formation affecting the artery or heart

Causes
- Age and family history
- Arteriosclerosis
- Cystic medial necrosis
- Infection
- Syphilis and other inflammatory disorders
- Trauma

Pathophysiologic changes

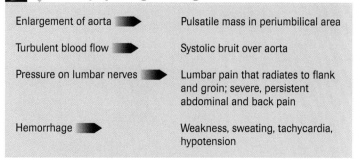

Enlargement of aorta ➡	Pulsatile mass in periumbilical area
Turbulent blood flow ➡	Systolic bruit over aorta
Pressure on lumbar nerves ➡	Lumbar pain that radiates to flank and groin; severe, persistent abdominal and back pain
Hemorrhage ➡	Weakness, sweating, tachycardia, hypotension

TYPES OF AORTIC ANEURYSMS

SACCULAR ANEURYSM

FUSIFORM ANEURYSM

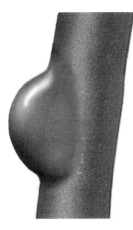
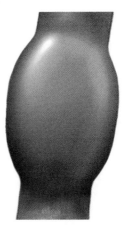

FALSE ANEURYSM

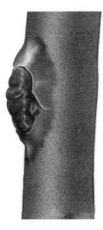

Aortic insufficiency

- Incomplete closure of aortic valve
- Usually results from scarring or retraction of valve leaflets

Causes

ACUTE AORTIC INSUFFICIENCY
- Acute ascending aortic dissection
- Chest trauma
- Endocarditis
- Prosthetic valve malfunction

CHRONIC AORTIC INSUFFICIENCY
- Ankylosing spondylitis
- Hypertension
- Marfan syndrome
- Rheumatic fever
- Syphilis
- Ventricular septal defect

Pathophysiologic changes

ACUTE AORTIC INSUFFICIENCY

Left ventricular failure ➤	Pulmonary congestion and shock

CHRONIC AORTIC INSUFFICIENCY

Increased pulmonary venous pressure and cardiac dysfunction ➤	Dyspnea, orthopnea, and paroxysmal nocturnal dyspnea
Left ventricular dysfunction ➤	Fatigue, exercise intolerance, pulmonary congestion, left-sided heart failure, pulsating nail beds, S_3
Inadequate coronary perfusion ➤	Angina
Hyperdynamic and tachycardic left ventricle ➤	Palpitations
Low diastolic pressure ➤	Widened pulse pressure
Regurgitant blood flow ➤	Diastolic blowing murmur at left sternal border

UNDERSTANDING AORTIC INSUFFICIENCY

NORMAL SEMILUNAR VALVE

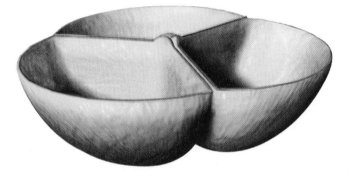

INSUFFICIENT SEMILUNAR VALVE

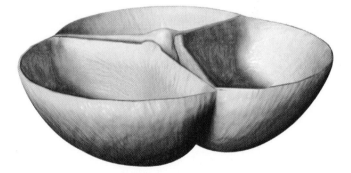

Aortic stenosis

- Narrowing of aortic valve
- Classified as acquired or rheumatic
- Classic triad of angina pectoris, syncope, and dyspnea

Causes
- Atherosclerosis
- Congenital aortic bicuspid valve
- Idiopathic fibrosis and calcification
- Rheumatic fever

Pathophysiologic changes

Abnormal diastolic function ➤	Exertional dyspnea
Increased oxygen requirement by myocardium and diminished oxygen delivery ➤	Angina
Systemic vasodilation or arrhythmias ➤	Syncope
Left-sided heart failure ➤	Pulmonary congestion
Forced blood flow across stenotic valve ➤	Harsh, rasping, crescendo-decrescendo systolic murmur

UNDERSTANDING AORTIC STENOSIS

NORMAL SEMILUNAR VALVE

STENOTIC SEMILUNAR VALVE

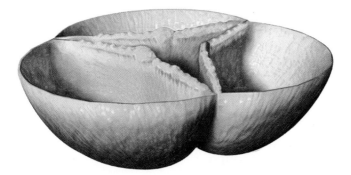

Atrial septal defect

- An acyanotic congenital heart defect that affects the flow of blood
- An abnormal opening between the left and right atria, shunting blood from the left atrium to the right atrium rather than from the left atrium to the left ventricle
- Results in ineffective pumping of the heart, increasing the risk of heart failure

Causes
- Unknown
- Associated with Down syndrome

Pathophysiologic changes

Decreased cardiac output ➤	Fatigue
Extra blood passing through the pulmonic valve ➤	Early- to mid-systolic murmur at the second or third intercostal space
Right heart volume overload ➤	Enlargement of the right atrium and right ventricular dilation
Mitral valve prolapse in older children ➤	Systolic click or late systolic murmur
Delayed closure of the pulmonic valve ➤	Split S_2

ATRIAL SEPTAL DEFECT

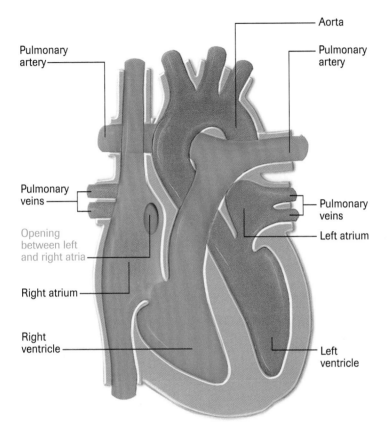

Aorta

Pulmonary artery

Pulmonary artery

Pulmonary veins

Pulmonary veins

Opening between left and right atria

Left atrium

Right atrium

Right ventricle

Left ventricle

Cardiac tamponade

- Rapid, unchecked rise in pressure in the pericardial sac resulting from blood or fluid accumulation
- Leads to compression of the heart and impaired diastolic filling, and limits cardiac output

Causes
- Acute myocardial infarction
- Chronic renal failure
- Connective tissue disorders
- Drug reaction
- Effusion
- Heparin or warfarin induced tamponade
- Idiopathic
- Pericarditis
- Postcardiac surgery
- Traumatic or nontraumatic hemorrhage

Pathophysiologic changes

Progressive fluid accumulation in the pericardial sac ➤	Compression of heart chambers
Ventricular obstruction and decreased ventricular filling ➤	Decreased cardiac output
Increased jugular pressure ➤	Elevated central venous pressure with jugular vein distention
Fluid in the pericardial sac ➤	Muffled heart sounds
Impaired diastolic filling ➤	Pulsus paradoxus

UNDERSTANDING CARDIAC TAMPONADE

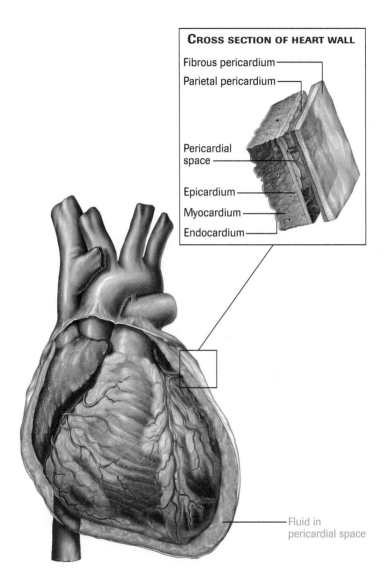

CROSS SECTION OF HEART WALL

Fibrous pericardium

Parietal pericardium

Pericardial space

Epicardium

Myocardium

Endocardium

Fluid in pericardial space

Cardiomyopathy, dilated

- Disease of heart muscle fibers
- Usually not diagnosed until advanced stage; prognosis generally poor

Causes
- Cardiotoxic effects of drug or alcohol
- Chemotherapy
- Drug hypersensitivity
- Hypertension
- Ischemic heart disease
- Peripartum syndrome related to toxemia
- Valvular disease
- Viral or bacterial infections

Pathophysiologic changes

Left-sided heart failure ➤	Shortness of breath, orthopnea, dyspnea, fatigue, dry cough at night
Right-sided heart failure ➤	Peripheral edema, hepatomegaly, jugular vein distention, weight gain
Low cardiac output ➤	Peripheral cyanosis, tachycardia
Mitral and tricuspid insufficiency ➤	Pansystolic murmur
Heart failure ➤	S_3 and S_4 gallop rhythms
Atrial fibrillation ➤	Irregular pulse
Decreased cardiac output ➤	Decreased renal perfusion

FEATURES OF DILATED CARDIOMYOPATHY

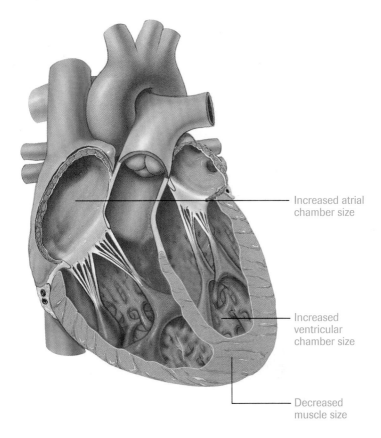

Increased atrial chamber size

Increased ventricular chamber size

Decreased muscle size

Cardiomyopathy, hypertrophic obstructive

- Primary disease of cardiac muscle
- Characterized by disproportionate, asymmetrical thickening of the interventricular septum and left ventricular hypertrophy
- Accounts for 50% of all sudden death cases in competitive athletes

Causes
- Autosomal dominant trait
- Hypertension
- Obstructive valvular disease
- Thyroid disease

Pathophysiologic changes

Mitral insufficiency ➤	Systolic ejection murmur along left sternal border and at apex
Inability of intramural coronary arteries to supply enough blood to meet increased oxygen demands of hypertrophied heart ➤	Angina
Arrhythmias or reduced ventricular filling leading to reduced cardiac output ➤	Syncope
Worsening of outflow tract obstruction from exercise-induced catecholamine releases ➤	Activity intolerance
Vigorous left ventricular contractions and early termination of left ventricular ejection ➤	Abrupt arterial pulse
Enlarged atrium ➤	Irregular pulse (atrial fibrillation)

FEATURES OF HYPERTROPHIC CARDIOMYOPATHY

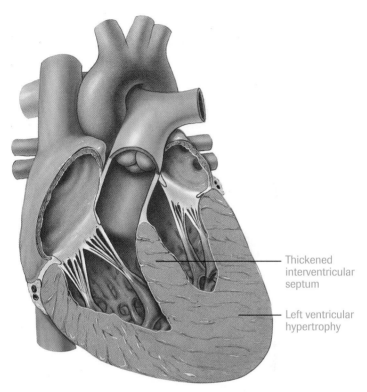

Thickened interventricular septum

Left ventricular hypertrophy

Cardiomyopathy, restrictive

- Disease of the heart muscle fibers
- Restricted ventricular filling due to decreased ventricular compliance and endocardial fibrosis and thickening
- Irreversible, if severe

Causes
- Amyloidosis
- Hemochromatosis
- Infiltrative neoplastic disease
- Sarcoidosis

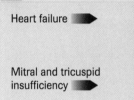 *Pathophysiologic changes*

Heart failure ➡	Fatigue, dyspnea, orthopnea, chest pain, edema, liver engorgement, peripheral cyanosis, pallor, and S_3 or S_4 gallop rhythms
Mitral and tricuspid insufficiency ➡	Systolic murmurs

FEATURES OF
RESTRICTIVE CARDIOMYOPATHY

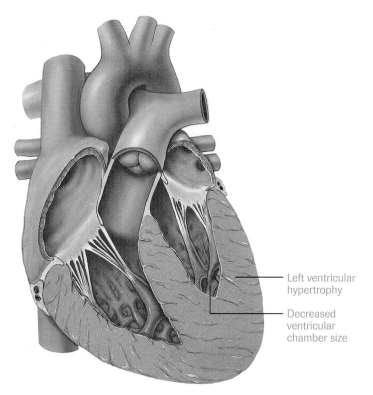

Left ventricular
hypertrophy

Decreased
ventricular
chamber size

Coarctation of the aorta

- Narrowing of the aorta, usually below the left subclavian artery at the site of the pulmonary artery joining the aorta
- Ostruction of blood flow that results in ineffective pumping of the heart and risk of heart failure
- Prognosis dependent on severity of associated cardiac anomalies

Causes
- Unknown
- May be associated with Turner's syndrome

Pathophysiologic changes

Heart failure ➤	Tachypnea, dyspnea, pulmonary edema, pallor, tachycardia, failure to thrive, cardiomegaly, and hepatomegaly
Reduced blood flow ➤	Claudication
Increased pressure in the arteries proximal to the coarctation ➤	Hypertension in the upper body
Restricted blood flow to the lower extremities ➤	Absent or diminished femoral pulses
Left to right shunting of blood ➤	Continuous midsystolic murmur

COARCTATION OF THE AORTA

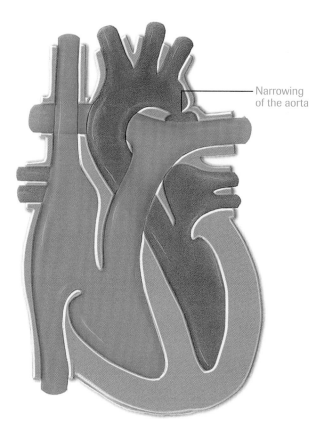

Narrowing
of the aorta

Coronary artery disease

- Results from a narrowing of the coronary arteries over time
- Leads to diminished supply of oxygen and nutrients to myocardial tissue from the decreased blood flow

Causes
- Atherosclerosis (most common)
- Congenital defects
- Dissecting aneurysm
- Infectious vasculitis
- Syphilis

Pathophysiologic changes

Arteries supplying the heart harden and narrow, causing a reduction in oxygen supply to myocardium ➤	Angina
Reflex stimulation of the vomiting centers by pain ➤	Nausea and vomiting
Sympathetic stimulation ➤	Cool extremities, diaphoresis and pallor

CORONARY ARTERY IN ATHEROSCLEROSIS

NORMAL CORONARY ARTERY

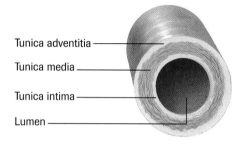

Tunica adventitia

Tunica media

Tunica intima

Lumen

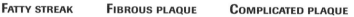

FATTY STREAK

FIBROUS PLAQUE

COMPLICATED PLAQUE

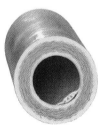
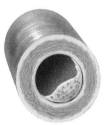
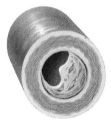

Deep vein thrombosis

- Characterized by inflammation and thrombus formation
- Usually refers to thrombosis in the deep veins of the legs
- Can progress and lead to pulmonary embolism
- Commonly begins with phlebitis, which provokes thrombus formation

Causes

- Accelerated blood clotting
- Endothelial damage
- Idiopathic
- Reduced blood flow, stasis

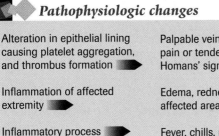 *Pathophysiologic changes*

Alteration in epithelial lining causing platelet aggregation, and thrombus formation ➤	Palpable vein, and lymphadenitis, pain or tenderness, positive Homans' sign
Inflammation of affected extremity ➤	Edema, redness and warmth over affected area
Inflammatory process ➤	Fever, chills, malaise

VENOUS THROMBUS

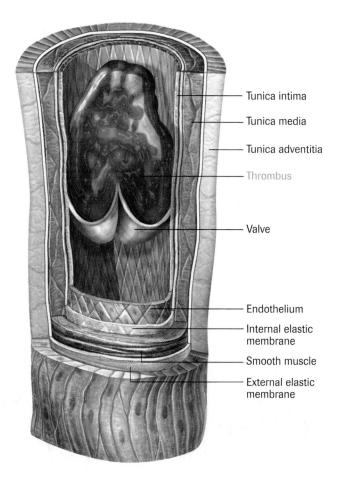

- Tunica intima
- Tunica media
- Tunica adventitia
- Thrombus
- Valve
- Endothelium
- Internal elastic membrane
- Smooth muscle
- External elastic membrane

Endocarditis

- Infection of the endocardium, heart valves, or cardiac prosthesis from bacteria or fungus
- May be caused by the introduction of bacteria into the bloodstream after a dental or urogenital procedure
- Risk factors: I.V. drug use, permanent central venous access lines, prior cardiac valve surgery, and weakened heart valves

Causes
- Bacteria (streptococci, staphylococci, enterococci, and gram-negative bacilli)
- Fungi (rare)

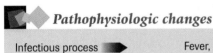
Pathophysiologic changes

Infectious process ➡	Fever, night sweats, chills
Infecting organisms cause vegetative growth on valves and heart lining leading to: Pulmonary infarction ➡	Cough, pleuritic pain, pleural friction rub, dyspnea, hemoptysis
Peripheral vascular occlusion ➡	Numbness and tingling in an arm, leg, finger, or toe
Valvular insufficiency ➡	Malaise, weakness, fatigue, weight loss, anorexia

TISSUE CHANGES IN ENDOCARDITIS

NORMAL HEART WALL

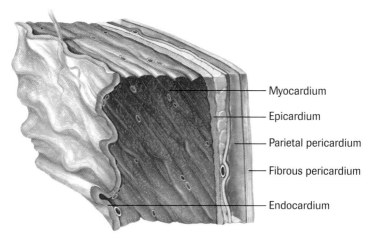

- Myocardium
- Epicardium
- Parietal pericardium
- Fibrous pericardium
- Endocardium

ENDOCARDITIS

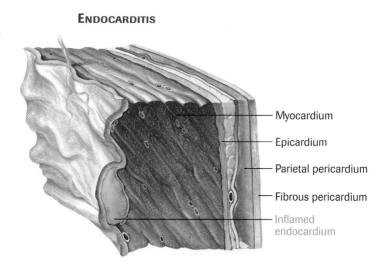

- Myocardium
- Epicardium
- Parietal pericardium
- Fibrous pericardium
- Inflamed endocardium

Heart failure

- Syndrome that occurs when heart can't pump enough blood to meet body's metabolic needs
- Results in intravascular and interstitial volume overload and poor tissue perfusion
- May be classified according to side of heart affected (left- or right-sided heart failure) or cardiac cycle involved (systolic or diastolic dysfunction)

Causes
- Abnormal cardiac muscle function
- Abnormal left ventricular volume, pressure, or filling

Pathophysiologic changes

LEFT-SIDED HEART FAILURE

Pulmonary congestion ➤	Dyspnea, orthopnea, paroxysmal nocturnal dyspnea, nonproductive cough, crackles
Reduced oxygenation; inability to increase cardiac output in the response to physical activity ➤	Fatigue
Left ventricular hypertrophy ➤	Point of the maximal impulse displaced toward left anterior axillary line
Sympathetic stimulation ➤	S_3
Atrial contraction against non-compliant ventricle ➤	S_4
Peripheral vasoconstriction ➤	Cool, pale skin

RIGHT-SIDED HEART FAILURE

Venous congestion ➤	Jugular vein distention, hepatomegaly
Congestion of liver and intestines ➤	Anorexia, fullness, and nausea
Fluid volume excess ➤	Weight gain, edema
Fluid retention ➤	Ascites or anasarca

WHAT HAPPENS IN HEART FAILURE

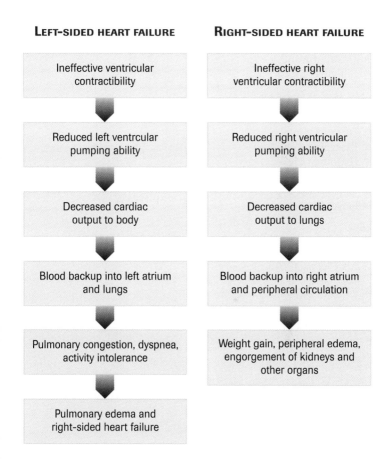

LEFT-SIDED HEART FAILURE

Ineffective ventricular contractibility

↓

Reduced left ventrcular pumping ability

↓

Decreased cardiac output to body

↓

Blood backup into left atrium and lungs

↓

Pulmonary congestion, dyspnea, activity intolerance

↓

Pulmonary edema and right-sided heart failure

RIGHT-SIDED HEART FAILURE

Ineffective right ventricular contractibility

↓

Reduced right ventricular pumping ability

↓

Decreased cardiac output to lungs

↓

Blood backup into right atrium and peripheral circulation

↓

Weight gain, peripheral edema, engorgement of kidneys and other organs

Hyperlipidemia

- Elevated lipids in the blood
- Lipids: cholesterol, cholesterol esters, phospholipids, and triglycerides
- Associated with premature coronary disease and peripheral vascular disease

Causes
PRIMARY CAUSE
- Inherited disorder

SECONDARY CAUSES
- Diabetes mellitus
- Dietary fat intake
- Excessive alcohol use
- Hypothyroidism
- Obesity
- Pancreatitis
- Renal disease

Pathophysiologic changes

Excessive lipids form plaques in blood vessels leading to:

Reduction in oxygen supply to myocardium ➤	Angina
Reflex stimulation of the vomiting centers by pain ➤	Nausea and vomiting
Sympathetic stimulation ➤	Cool extremities, diaphoresis, and pallor
Hypercholesterolemia ➤	Xanthomas

UNDERSTANDING HYPERLIPIDEMIA

CHOLESTEROL TRANSPORT IN THE BLOOD

Lipoproteins act as "fat shuttles," transporting cholesterol through the bloodstream.

Very-low-density lipoprotein (VLDL) travels through the bloodstream, attaching to the lining of the capillaries. There, its fatty core of cholesterol is drawn out.

Red blood cell

Capillary

VLDL

HDL

IDL

LDL

HOW CHOLESTEROL IS MADE

The small particles of intermediate-density lipoprotein (IDL) that remain in the blood shed tiny disklike particles of high-density lipoprotein (HDL; good cholesterol).

Low-density lipoprotein (LDL; bad cholesterol) remains in the blood and travels back to the liver to be removed.

Food particles

Liver

Intestine

Chylomicron

Breakdown of triglyceride

Breakdown of triglyceride

Free fatty acids

Hypertension

- Intermittent or sustained elevation of systolic blood pressure
- Two major types: essential (primary) hypertension and secondary hypertension

Causes
PRIMARY HYPERTENSION
- Unknown
- Risk factors: advancing age, family history, lifestyle, race, sleep apnea

SECONDARY HYPERTENSION
- Brain tumor, head injury, and tetraplegia
- Cocaine, epoetin alfa, estrogen replacement therapy, monoamine oxidase inhibitors taken with tyramine, nonsteroidal anti-inflammatory drugs, oral contraceptives, and sympathetic stimulants
- Cushing's syndrome; hyperaldosteronism and thyroid, pituitary, or parathyroid dysfunction; pheochromocytoma
- Parenchymal disease and renal artery stenosis

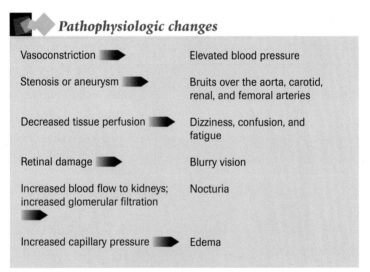

Pathophysiologic changes

Vasoconstriction ➤	Elevated blood pressure
Stenosis or aneurysm ➤	Bruits over the aorta, carotid, renal, and femoral arteries
Decreased tissue perfusion ➤	Dizziness, confusion, and fatigue
Retinal damage ➤	Blurry vision
Increased blood flow to kidneys; increased glomerular filtration ➤	Nocturia
Increased capillary pressure ➤	Edema

BLOOD VESSEL DAMAGE IN HYPERTENSION

Increased intra-arterial pressure damages the endothelium.

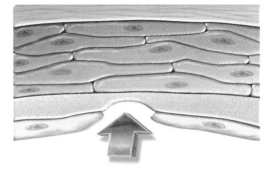

Angiotensin II induces endothelial wall contraction, allowing plasma to leak through inter-endothelial spaces.

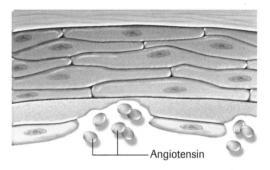

Angiotensin

Plasma constituents deposited in the vessel wall cause medial necrosis.

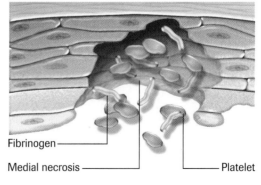

Fibrinogen

Medial necrosis

Platelet

Mitral insufficiency

- Inadequate closing of mitral value
- Backflow of blood from left ventricle to the right atrium during systole

Causes
- Hypertrophic obstructive cardiomyopathy
- Mitral valve prolapse
- Myocardial infarction
- Rheumatic fever
- Ruptured chordae tendineae
- Transposition of great arteries

Pathophysiologic changes

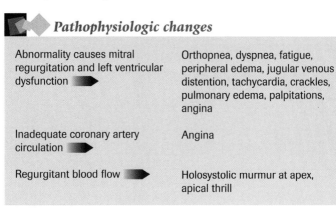

Abnormality causes mitral regurgitation and left ventricular dysfunction ➡ Orthopnea, dyspnea, fatigue, peripheral edema, jugular venous distention, tachycardia, crackles, pulmonary edema, palpitations, angina

Inadequate coronary artery circulation ➡ Angina

Regurgitant blood flow ➡ Holosystolic murmur at apex, apical thrill

UNDERSTANDING MITRAL INSUFFICIENCY

NORMAL ATRIOVENTRICULAR VALVE

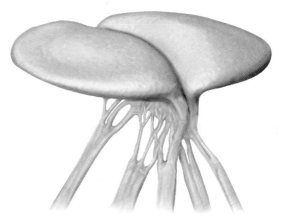

INSUFFICIENT ATRIOVENTRICULAR VALVE

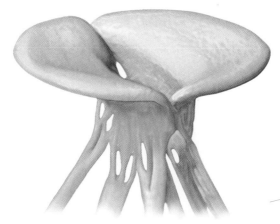

Mitral stenosis

- Narrowing of the mitral valve orifice
- Valve leaflets thickened by fibrosis and calcification

Causes

- Adverse effect of fenfluramine and phentermine diet drug combination
- Atrial myxoma
- Congenital abnormalities
- Endocarditis
- Rheumatic fever

Pathophysiologic changes

Cardiac dysfunction ➤	Dyspnea on exertion, paroxysmal nocturnal dyspnea, orthopnea, weakness, fatigue, and palpitations
Heart failure ➤	Peripheral edema, jugular venous distention, hepatomegaly, tachycardia, crackles, pulmonary edema
Turbulent blood flow over stenotic valve ➤	Opening snap and diastolic murmur

UNDERSTANDING MITRAL STENOSIS

Normal atrioventricular valve

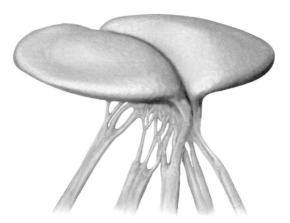

Stenotic atrioventricular valve

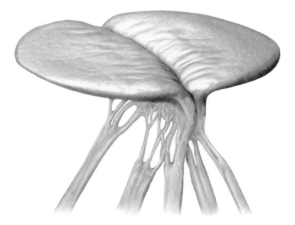

Mitral valve prolapse

- Billowing and improper closure of the mitral valve
- Occurs more frequently in women than men

Causes
- Autosomal dominant inheritance
- Genetic or environmental interruption of valve development during week 5 or 6 of gestation
- Inherited connective tissue disorders, such as Ehlers-Danlos syndrome, Marfan syndrome, and osteogenesis imperfecta

Pathophysiologic changes

Blood regurgitation from the left ventricle back into the left atrium	Dizziness, syncope, palpitation, chest pain, murmur
Atrial or ventricular arrhythmias	Palpitations
Commonly produces no symptoms	

VALVE POSITION IN MITRAL VALVE PROLAPSE

CROSS SECTION OF LEFT VENTRICLE

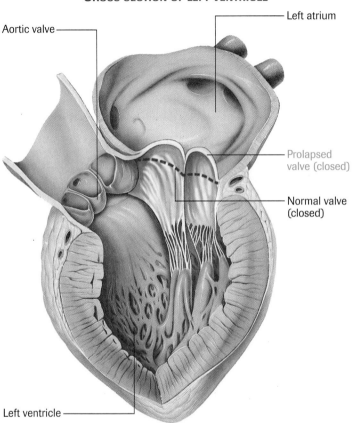

Left atrium

Aortic valve

Prolapsed valve (closed)

Normal valve (closed)

Left ventricle

Myocardial infarction

- Form of acute coronary artery syndrome
- Reduced blood flow through one or more coronary arteries initiating myocardial ischemia and necrosis

Causes
- Coronary artery stenosis and spasm
- Drug use, especially amphetamines and cocaine
- Thrombosis

Pathophysiologic changes

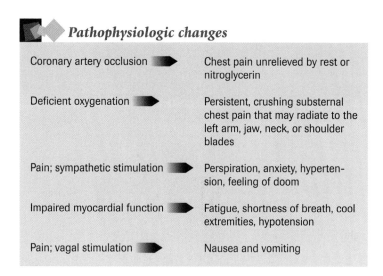

Coronary artery occlusion ➤	Chest pain unrelieved by rest or nitroglycerin
Deficient oxygenation ➤	Persistent, crushing substernal chest pain that may radiate to the left arm, jaw, neck, or shoulder blades
Pain; sympathetic stimulation ➤	Perspiration, anxiety, hypertension, feeling of doom
Impaired myocardial function ➤	Fatigue, shortness of breath, cool extremities, hypotension
Pain; vagal stimulation ➤	Nausea and vomiting

TISSUE DESTRUCTION IN MYOCARDIAL INFARCTION

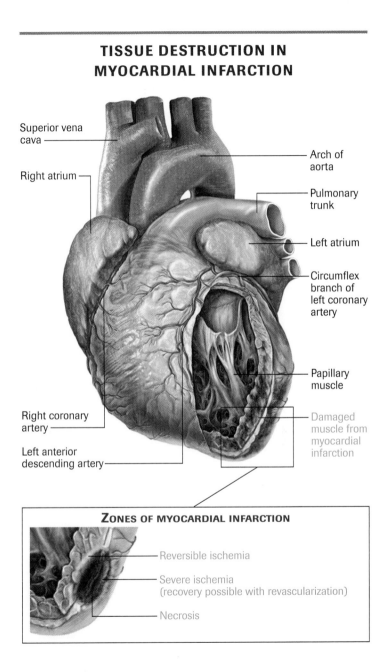

Superior vena cava

Arch of aorta

Right atrium

Pulmonary trunk

Left atrium

Circumflex branch of left coronary artery

Papillary muscle

Right coronary artery

Damaged muscle from myocardial infarction

Left anterior descending artery

ZONES OF MYOCARDIAL INFARCTION

Reversible ischemia

Severe ischemia (recovery possible with revascularization)

Necrosis

Myocarditis

- Focal or diffuse inflammation of the cardiac muscle
- May be acute or chronic and can occur at any age
- Typically doesn't manifest cardiovascular symptoms or electrocardiogram changes

Causes

- Chemotherapeutic agents or radiation therapy
- Chronic alcoholism
- Hypersensitive immune reactions
- Infections
- Systemic autoimmune disorders
- Toxins, such as chemicals, cocaine, or lead

Pathophysiologic changes

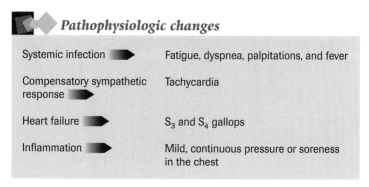

Systemic infection ➤	Fatigue, dyspnea, palpitations, and fever
Compensatory sympathetic response ➤	Tachycardia
Heart failure ➤	S_3 and S_4 gallops
Inflammation ➤	Mild, continuous pressure or soreness in the chest

TISSUE CHANGES IN MYOCARDITIS

NORMAL HEART WALL

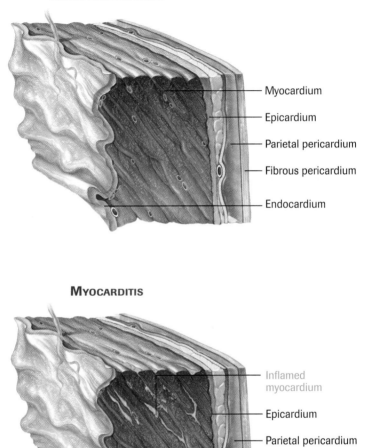

Myocardium

Epicardium

Parietal pericardium

Fibrous pericardium

Endocardium

MYOCARDITIS

Inflamed myocardium

Epicardium

Parietal pericardium

Fibrous pericardium

Endocardium

Patent ductus arteriosus

- Lumen of the ductus arteriosus remaining open after birth instead of closing
- Left-to-right shunt of blood from the aorta to the pulmonary artery resulting in recirculation of arterial blood through the lungs
- Fatal condition without surgical repair

Causes

- Coarctation of the aorta
- Living at high altitudes
- Premature birth
- Pulmonary and aortic stenosis
- Rubella syndrome
- Ventricular septal defect

Pathophysiologic changes

Increased volume of blood shunting through the lungs and increased cardiac workload ➡	Respiratory distress with heart failure in infants
Shunting of blood from the aorta to the pulmonary artery throughout systole and diastole ➡	Gibson murmur
Left ventricular hypertrophy ➡	Prominent left ventricular impulse
Elevated systolic blood pressure ➡	Widened pulse pressure
Heart failure ➡	Slow motor development, failure to thrive

PATENT DUCTUS ARTERIOSUS

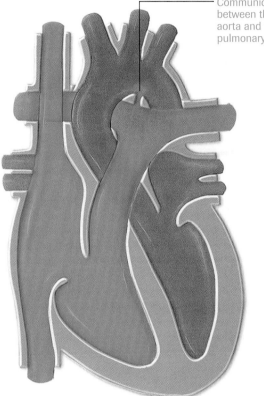

Communication between the aorta and the pulmonary artery

Pericarditis

- Inflammation of pericardium
- Can be fibrous or effusive, with purulent, serous, or hemorrhagic exudates (acute)
- Characterized by dense, fibrous pericardial thickening (chronic)

Causes
- Autoimmune or hypersensitivity disease
- Bacterial, fungal, or viral infection
- Cardiac injury, cardiac surgery
- Drugs, such as hydralazine or procainamide
- High-dose radiation to chest
- Idiopathic
- Neoplasms
- Uremia

Pathophysiologic changes

Roughened, inflamed, irritated pericardial membranes ➡	Pericardial friction rub; sharp, often sudden pain, starting over the sternum and radiating to the neck, shoulders, back, and arms
Pleuritic pain ➡	Shallow, rapid respirations
Inflammation ➡	Mild fever
Pericardial effusion ➡	Dyspnea, orthopnea, and tachycardia
Fluid accumulation ➡	Muffled and distant heart sounds
Increased systemic venous pressure ➡	Fluid retention, ascites, hepatomegaly, jugular vein distention, and signs of chronic right-sided heart failure

TISSUE CHANGES IN PERICARDITIS

NORMAL HEART WALL

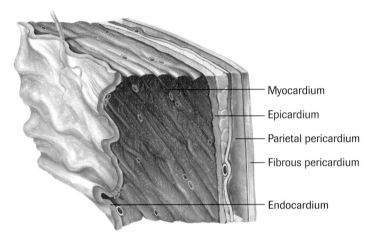

- Myocardium
- Epicardium
- Parietal pericardium
- Fibrous pericardium
- Endocardium

PERICARDITIS

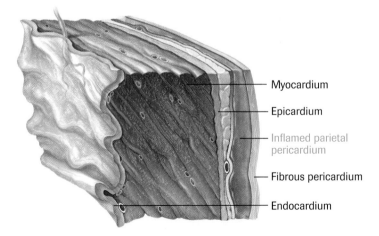

- Myocardium
- Epicardium
- Inflamed parietal pericardium
- Fibrous pericardium
- Endocardium

Pulmonic stenosis

- Narrowing of the pulmonic valve orifice
- Obstructed right ventricular outflow causing right ventricular hypertrophy
- Results in right-sided heart failure
- Associated with tetralogy of Fallot
- Commonly produces no symptoms

Causes
- Congenital stenosis of valve cusp
- Rheumatic fever (rare)

Pathophysiologic changes

Right-sided heart failure ➡	Dyspnea on exertion, chest pain, syncope, fatigue, jugular vein distention
Stenotic valve cusp ➡	Systolic murmur at the left sternal border, S_2 split

UNDERSTANDING PULMONIC STENOSIS

NORMAL SEMILUNAR VALVE

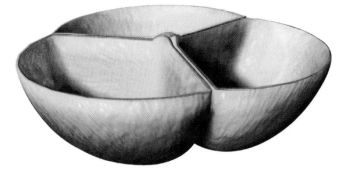

STENOTIC SEMILUNAR VALVE

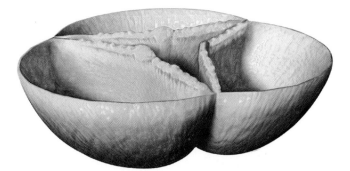

Raynaud's disease

- Arteriospastic disorder affecting the hands and occasionally the feet
- Characterized by vasospasms in small peripheral arteries and arterioles
- Response to cold exposure or stress

Causes
- Unknown
- Family history

Pathophysiologic changes

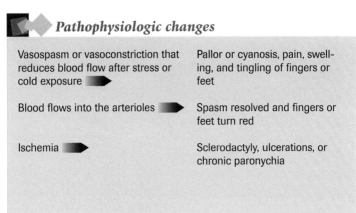

Vasospasm or vasoconstriction that reduces blood flow after stress or cold exposure ➤	Pallor or cyanosis, pain, swelling, and tingling of fingers or feet
Blood flows into the arterioles ➤	Spasm resolved and fingers or feet turn red
Ischemia ➤	Sclerodactyly, ulcerations, or chronic paronychia

PROGRESSIVE VASCULAR CHANGES IN RAYNAUD'S DISEASE

PALLOR DUE TO DECREASED OR ABSENT BLOOD FLOW

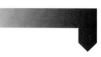

CYANOSIS DUE TO CAPILLARY DILATION

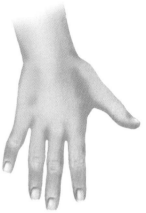

RUBOR DUE TO EXCESSIVE HYPEREMIA RESULTING FROM REACTIVE VASODILATION

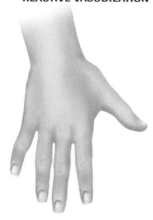

Rheumatic heart disease

- Systemic inflammatory disease of childhood
- Refers to the cardiac manifestations of rheumatic fever and includes pancarditis in early phase and chronic valvular disease in late phase
- Involves heart, joints, central nervous system, skin, and subcutaneous tissues

Causes

- Group-A beta-hemolytic streptococcal pharyngitis

Pathophysiologic changes

Hypersensitivity reaction ➤	Erythema marginatum, a nonpruritic macular, transient rash on the trunk or inner aspects of the upper arm or thighs, leading to red lesions with blanched centers
Inflammatory and infectious processes ➤	Fever, polyarthritis, joint pain, and swelling and redness of joints
Endocarditis ➤	Valve leaflet swelling, erosion along the line of leaflet closure, and vegetation
Carditis ➤	Development of subcutaneous nodules near tendons or bony prominences in joints

SEQUELAE OF RHEUMATIC HEART DISEASE

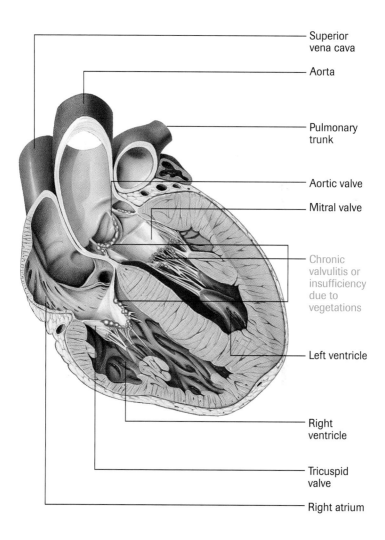

Superior vena cava

Aorta

Pulmonary trunk

Aortic valve

Mitral valve

Chronic valvulitis or insufficiency due to vegetations

Left ventricle

Right ventricle

Tricuspid valve

Right atrium

Shock, cardiogenic

- Diminished cardiac output that severely impairs tissue perfusion
- Also known as *pump failure*

Causes
- Acute mitral or aortic insufficiency
- End-stage cardiomyopathy
- Myocardial infarction
- Myocardial ischemia
- Myocarditis
- Papillary muscle dysfunction
- Ventricular aneurysm
- Ventricular septal defect

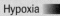 *Pathophysiologic changes*

Sympathetic stimulation ▶	Tachycardia, bounding pulse
Cerebral hypoxia ▶	Restlessness, irritability, tachypnea
Vasoconstriction ▶	Reduced urine output; cool, pale skin
Failure of compensatory mechanisms ▶	Hypotension
Reduced stroke volume, decreased cardiac output ▶	Narrowed pulse pressure; weak, rapid, thready pulse
Poor renal perfusion ▶	Reduced urine output
Hypoxia ▶	Cyanosis
Reduced cerebral perfusion, acid base imbalance, or electrolyte abnormalities ▶	Unconsciousness and absent reflexes
Weakening of patient; respiratory center depression ▶	Slow, shallow, or Cheyne-Stokes respirations

WHAT HAPPENS IN CARDIOGENIC SHOCK

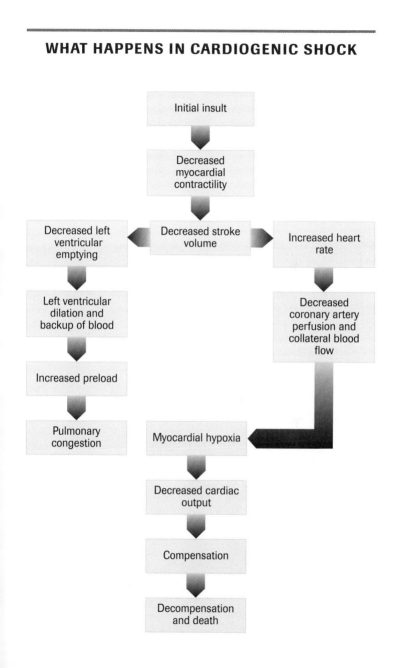

Shock, hypovolemic

- Reduced intravascular blood volume causing circulatory dysfunction and inadequate tissue perfusion
- Requires early recognition and prompt treatment to improve prognosis

Causes
- Ascites
- Blood loss
- Burns
- Fluid shifts
- GI fluid loss
- Hemothorax
- Peritonitis
- Renal loss

Pathophysiologic changes

Sympathetic stimulation ➤	Tachycardia
Cerebral hypoxia ➤	Restlessness, irritability, and tachypnea
Reduced fluid volume; vasoconstriction ➤	Reduced urine output; cool, pale, clammy skin
Failure of compensatory mechanisms ➤	Hypotension
Reduced stroke volume; decreased cardiac output ➤	Narrowed pulse pressure; weak, rapid, thready pulse
Weakening of patient ➤	Shallow respirations
Poor renal perfusion ➤	Reduced urine output
Hypoxia ➤	Cyanosis
Tissue anoxia ➤	Metabolic acidosis

WHAT HAPPENS IN HYPOVOLEMIC SHOCK

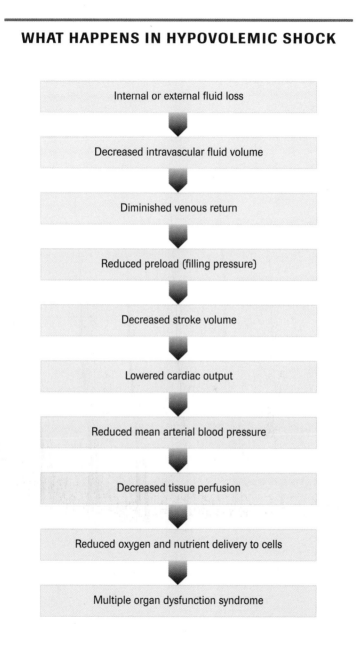

Internal or external fluid loss

↓

Decreased intravascular fluid volume

↓

Diminished venous return

↓

Reduced preload (filling pressure)

↓

Decreased stroke volume

↓

Lowered cardiac output

↓

Reduced mean arterial blood pressure

↓

Decreased tissue perfusion

↓

Reduced oxygen and nutrient delivery to cells

↓

Multiple organ dysfunction syndrome

Shock, septic

- Inadequate tissue perfusion, metabolic changes, and circulatory collapse as response to infection
- Develops in 25% of patients with gram-negative bacteremia

Causes
- Gram-negative bacteria
- Gram-positive bacteria

Pathophysiologic changes

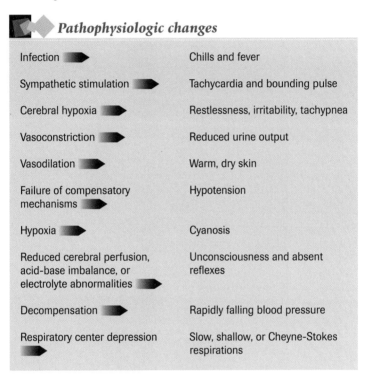

Infection ➤	Chills and fever
Sympathetic stimulation ➤	Tachycardia and bounding pulse
Cerebral hypoxia ➤	Restlessness, irritability, tachypnea
Vasoconstriction ➤	Reduced urine output
Vasodilation ➤	Warm, dry skin
Failure of compensatory mechanisms ➤	Hypotension
Hypoxia ➤	Cyanosis
Reduced cerebral perfusion, acid-base imbalance, or electrolyte abnormalities ➤	Unconsciousness and absent reflexes
Decompensation ➤	Rapidly falling blood pressure
Respiratory center depression ➤	Slow, shallow, or Cheyne-Stokes respirations

WHAT HAPPENS IN SEPTIC SHOCK

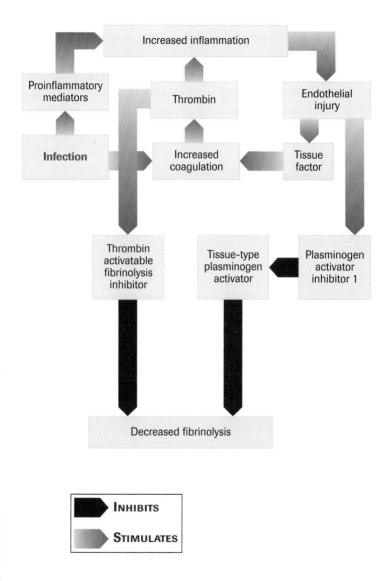

Tetralogy of Fallot

- Combination of four cardiac defects: ventricular septal defect (VSD), right ventricular outflow tract obstruction, right ventricular hypertrophy, and an aorta positioned above the VSD (dextroposition of the aorta)
- Abnormal blood shunting that results in mixing of unoxygenated blood with oxygenated blood
- May coexist with other congenital acyanotic heart defects

Causes
- Fetal alcohol syndrome
- Thalidomide use during pregnancy

Pathophysiologic changes

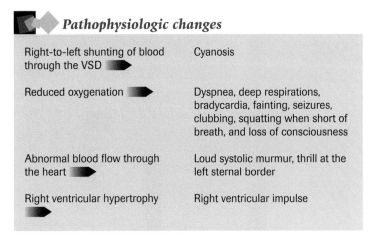

Right-to-left shunting of blood through the VSD ➡	Cyanosis
Reduced oxygenation ➡	Dyspnea, deep respirations, bradycardia, fainting, seizures, clubbing, squatting when short of breath, and loss of consciousness
Abnormal blood flow through the heart ➡	Loud systolic murmur, thrill at the left sternal border
Right ventricular hypertrophy ➡	Right ventricular impulse

UNDERSTANDING TETRALOGY OF FALLOT

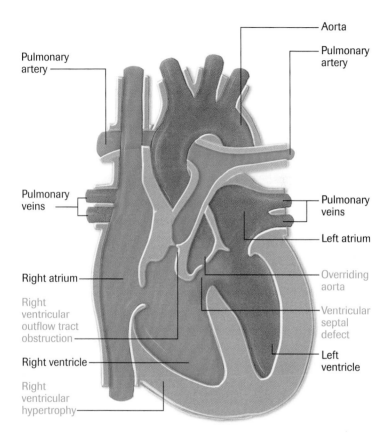

Aorta

Pulmonary artery

Pulmonary artery

Pulmonary veins

Pulmonary veins

Left atrium

Right atrium

Overriding aorta

Right ventricular outflow tract obstruction

Ventricular septal defect

Right ventricle

Left ventricle

Right ventricular hypertrophy

Transposition of the great arteries

- Cyanotic congenital heart defect
- Reversed great arteries: aorta arising from the right ventricle and pulmonary artery from the left ventricle
- Produces two noncommunicating circulatory systems: pulmonic and systemic

Causes
- Unknown

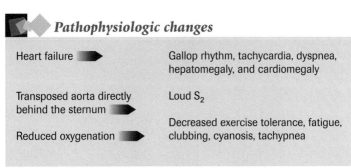

Pathophysiologic changes

Heart failure	Gallop rhythm, tachycardia, dyspnea, hepatomegaly, and cardiomegaly
Transposed aorta directly behind the sternum	Loud S_2
Reduced oxygenation	Decreased exercise tolerance, fatigue, clubbing, cyanosis, tachypnea

TRANSPOSITION OF THE GREAT ARTERIES

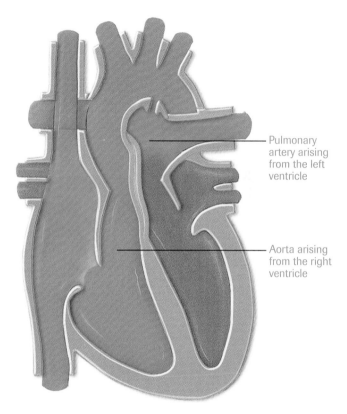

Pulmonary artery arising from the left ventricle

Aorta arising from the right ventricle

___ Ventricular septal defect ___

- Most common acyanotic congenital heart disorder
- Opening in the septum between the ventricles allowing blood to shunt between the left and right ventricles
- Ineffective pumping of the heart and risk for heart failure

Causes
- Down syndrome and other autosomal trisomies
- Fetal alcohol syndrome
- Patent ductus arteriosus and coarctation of the aorta
- Prematurity
- Renal anomalies

Pathophysiologic changes

Abnormal blood flow through the ventricular septal defect ➤	Loud, harsh systolic murmur and palpable thrill
Increased pressure gradient across the ventricular septal defect ➤	Loud, widely split pulmonic component of S_2
Hypertrophy of the heart ➤	Displacement of the point of maximal impulse

VENTRICULAR SEPTAL DEFECT

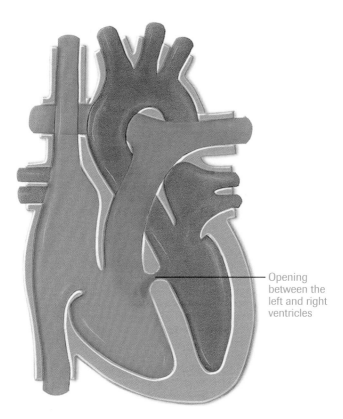

Opening between the left and right ventricles

2

Respiratory system

Acute respiratory distress syndrome

- Form of noncardiogenic pulmonary edema that can quickly lead to acute respiratory failure
- Also known as *shock lung, stiff lung, white lung, wet lung*
- If not promptly diagnosed and treated, may lead to death within 48 hours

Causes
- Anaphylaxis
- Aspiration of gastric contents
- Diffuse pneumonia
- Drug overdose
- Idiosyncratic drug reaction
- Indirect or direct lung trauma
- Inhalation of noxious gases
- Near drowning
- Oxygen toxicity
- Sepsis

Pathophysiologic changes

Decreasing oxygen levels in blood (hypoxemia)	Tachycardia; rapid, shallow breathing; dyspnea
Hypoxemia effects on pneumotaxic center	Increased rate of ventilation
Increased effort required to expand stiff lung	Intercostal and suprasternal retractions
Fluid accumulation in lungs	Crackles and rhonchi
Hypoxic brain cells	Restlessness, apprehension, mental sluggishness, and motor dysfunction
Accumulation of carbon dioxide in blood (hypercarbia)	Respiratory acidosis
Failure of compensatory mechanisms	Hypoxemia, metabolic acidosis

ALVEOLAR CHANGES IN ACUTE RESPIRATORY DISTRESS SYNDROME

Phase 1. Injury reduces normal blood flow to the lungs. Platelets aggregate and release histamine, serotonin, and bradykinin.

Phase 2. Those substances, especially histamine, inflame and damage the alveolocapillary membrane, increasing capillary permeability. Fluids then shift into the interstitial space.

Phase 3. As capillary permeability increases, proteins and fluids leak out, increasing interstitial osmotic pressure and causing pulmonary edema.

Phase 4. Decreased blood flow and fluids in the alveoli damage surfactant and impair the cell's ability to produce more. As a result, alveoli collapse, impeding gas exchange and decreasing lung compliance.

Phase 5. Sufficient oxygen can't cross the alveolocapillary membrane, but carbon dioxide (CO_2) can and is lost with every exhalation. Oxygen (O_2) and CO_2 levels decrease in the blood.

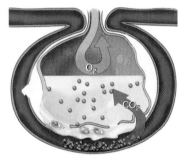

Phase 6. Pulmonary edema worsens, inflammation leads to fibrosis, and gas exchange is further impeded.

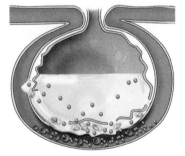

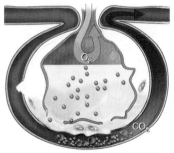

Asthma

- Chronic inflammatory airway disorder characterized by airflow obstruction and airway hyperresponsiveness to multiplicity of stimuli
- Type of chronic obstructive pulmonary disease
- May result from sensitivity to extrinsic or intrinsic allergens

Causes

- Extrinsic asthma: pollen, animal dander, house dust or mold, kapok or feather pillows, food additive containing sulfites, other sensitizing substances
- Intrinsic asthma: irritants, emotional stress, fatigue, endocrine changes, temperature variations, humidity variations, exposure to noxious fumes, anxiety, coughing or laughing, genetic factors

Pathophysiologic changes

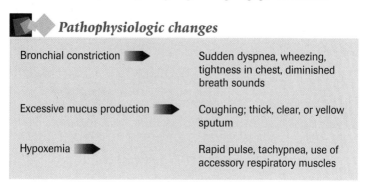

Bronchial constriction ➡	Sudden dyspnea, wheezing, tightness in chest, diminished breath sounds
Excessive mucus production ➡	Coughing; thick, clear, or yellow sputum
Hypoxemia ➡	Rapid pulse, tachypnea, use of accessory respiratory muscles

ASTHMATIC BRONCHUS

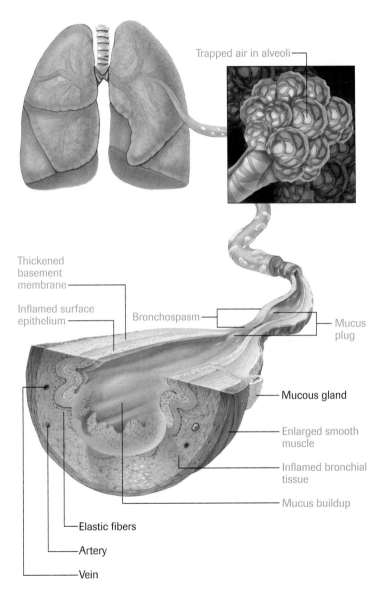

Trapped air in alveoli

Thickened basement membrane

Inflamed surface epithelium

Bronchospasm

Mucus plug

Mucous gland

Enlarged smooth muscle

Inflamed bronchial tissue

Mucus buildup

Elastic fibers

Artery

Vein

Chronic bronchitis

- Form of chronic obstructive pulmonary disease
- Characterized by excessive production of tracheobronchial mucus and chronic cough (at least 3 months each year for 2 consecutive years)
- Distinguishing characteristic: airflow obstruction

Causes
- Cigarette smoking
- Genetic predisposition
- Organic or inorganic dusts and noxious gas exposure
- Respiratory tract infection

Pathophysiologic changes

Hypersecretion of goblet cells ➤	Copious gray, white, or yellow sputum and productive cough
Obstruction of airflow to lower bronchial tree ➤	Dyspnea
Hypoxia ➤	Tachypnea, cyanosis, and use of accessory muscles for breathing
Narrow, mucus-filled respiratory passages ➤	Wheezing and rhonchi
Compensatory mechanism to maintain patent airway ➤	Prolonged expiratory time

MUCUS BUILDUP IN CHRONIC BRONCHITIS

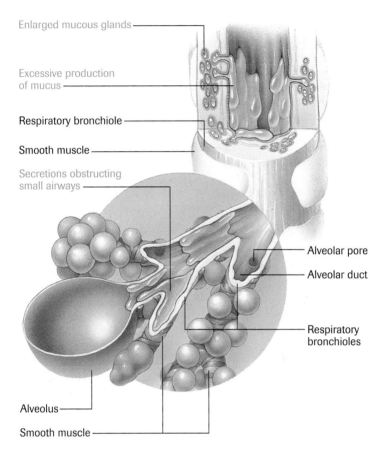

Enlarged mucous glands

Excessive production of mucus

Respiratory bronchiole

Smooth muscle

Secretions obstructing small airways

Alveolar pore

Alveolar duct

Respiratory bronchioles

Alveolus

Smooth muscle

Emphysema

- Form of chronic obstructive pulmonary disease
- Characterized by abnormal, permanent enlargement of acini accompanied by destruction of alveolar walls
- Airflow limitation caused by lack of elastic recoil in lungs

Causes
- Alpha$_1$–antitrypsin deficiency
- Cigarette smoking
- Recurrent inflammation of lungs

Pathophysiologic changes

Decreased oxygenation ➤	Tachypnea, dyspnea on exertion
Overdistention and over-inflation of lungs ➤	Barrel-shaped chest
Accessory muscle use ➤	Prolonged expiration, grunting, pursed-lip breathing
Trapped air in alveolar space; alveolar wall destruction ➤	Decreased breath sounds and tactile fremitus, hyperresonance on chest percussion
Chronic hypoxia ➤	Clubbed fingers and toes
Hypoventilation ➤	Decreased chest expansion
Bronchiolar collapse ➤	Crackles and wheezing on inspiration

LUNG CHANGES IN EMPHYSEMA

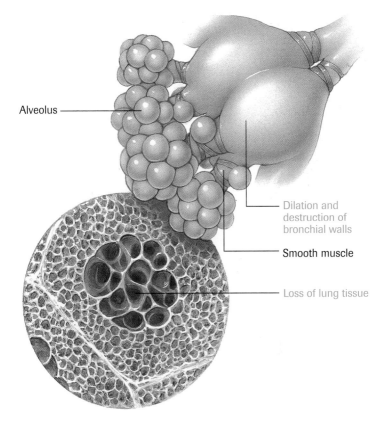

Alveolus

Dilation and destruction of bronchial walls

Smooth muscle

Loss of lung tissue

Fat embolism syndrome

- Traumatic release of fat droplets that act as emboli and become impacted in the microvasculature
- Rare but potentially fatal disorder
- Involves pulmonary, cerebral, and cutaneous manifestations and occurs 24 to 48 hours postinjury

Causes

- Fractures of the femur, pelvis, ribs, or tibia
- Orthopedic surgery

Pathophysiologic changes

Decreased pulmonary circulation and hypoxemia ➤	Dyspnea, increased respiratory rate, accessory muscle use, mental status changes
Altered platelet function ➤	Thrombocytopenia, petechiae and, possibly, disseminated intravascular coagulation
Increased workload of the right side of the heart ➤	Pulmonary edema

HOW FAT EMBOLISM THREATENS PULMONARY CIRCULATION

Bone injury

Bone marrow from a fractured bone releases fat globules.

Fat globules enter the pulmonary circulation, where they form emboli that block pulmonary circulation.

Alveolus

Capillary permeability is increased and lung surfactant is inactivated, allowing protein-rich fluid to leak into the alveoli, causing pulmonary edema.

Idiopathic pulmonary fibrosis

- Chronic and usually fatal interstitial disease
- Associated with inflammation and fibrosis
- Once a rare disorder, now more frequently diagnosed
- Survival after diagnosis generally 3 to 5 years

Causes
- Inflammatory, immune, and fibrotic processes in the lung

Pathophysiologic changes

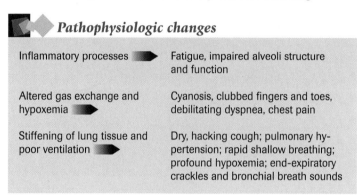

Inflammatory processes ➤	Fatigue, impaired alveoli structure and function
Altered gas exchange and hypoxemia ➤	Cyanosis, clubbed fingers and toes, debilitating dyspnea, chest pain
Stiffening of lung tissue and poor ventilation ➤	Dry, hacking cough; pulmonary hypertension; rapid shallow breathing; profound hypoxemia; end-expiratory crackles and bronchial breath sounds

END-STAGE FIBROSIS

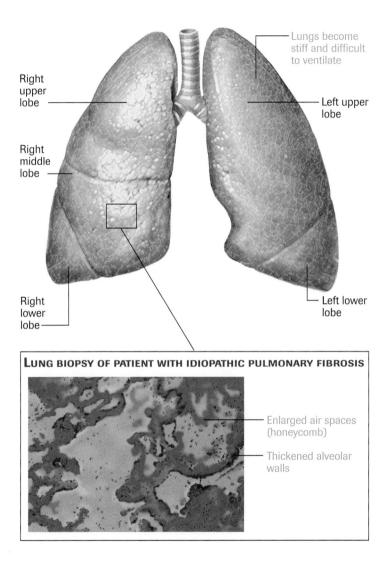

Lungs become stiff and difficult to ventilate

Right upper lobe

Left upper lobe

Right middle lobe

Right lower lobe

Left lower lobe

LUNG BIOPSY OF PATIENT WITH IDIOPATHIC PULMONARY FIBROSIS

Enlarged air spaces (honeycomb)

Thickened alveolar walls

Lung cancer

- Development of neoplasm, usually within wall or epithelium of bronchial tree
- Most common types: epidermoid (squamous cell) carcinoma, small cell (oat cell) carcinoma, adenocarcinoma, and large cell (anaplastic) carcinoma

Causes
- Cigarette smoking
- Genetic predisposition
- Inhalation of carcinogenic and industrial air pollutants

Pathophysiologic changes

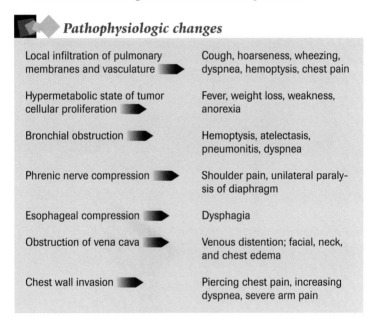

Local infiltration of pulmonary membranes and vasculature ➡	Cough, hoarseness, wheezing, dyspnea, hemoptysis, chest pain
Hypermetabolic state of tumor cellular proliferation ➡	Fever, weight loss, weakness, anorexia
Bronchial obstruction ➡	Hemoptysis, atelectasis, pneumonitis, dyspnea
Phrenic nerve compression ➡	Shoulder pain, unilateral paralysis of diaphragm
Esophageal compression ➡	Dysphagia
Obstruction of vena cava ➡	Venous distention; facial, neck, and chest edema
Chest wall invasion ➡	Piercing chest pain, increasing dyspnea, severe arm pain

TUMOR INFILTRATION IN LUNG CANCER

RIGHT LUNG—ANTERIOR VIEW

Trachea

Metastasis to hilar lymph nodes

Bronchus

Tumor projecting into bronchi

Metastasis to carinal lymph nodes

BRONCHOSCOPIC VIEW

Tumor projecting into bronchi

Pleural effusion

- Excess of fluid in the pleural space
- Increased production or inadequate removal of excess fluid resulting in transudative or exudative pleural effusion
- Empyema due to the accumulation of pus and necrotic tissue in the pleural space

Causes
TRANSUDATIVE PLEURAL EFFUSION
- Disorders causing expanded intravascular volume
- Heart failure
- Hepatic disease with ascites
- Hypoalbuminemia
- Peritoneal dialysis

EXUDATIVE PLEURAL EFFUSION
- Bacterial or fungal pneumonitis or empyema
- Chest trauma
- Collagen disease such as systemic lupus erythematosus
- Malignancy
- Myxedema
- Pancreatitis
- Pulmonary embolism with or without infarction
- Subphrenic abscess
- Tuberculosis

EMPYEMA
- Carcinoma
- Esophageal rupture
- Idiopathic infection
- Perforation
- Pneumonitis

Pathophysiologic changes

Fluid movement into the pleural space ➡	Decreased breath sounds; dullness over the effused areas; pleuritic chest pain; dyspnea; displaced point of maximum impulse, based on size of effusion
Inflammatory process ➡	Fever, malaise

LUNG COMPRESSION IN PLEURAL EFFUSION

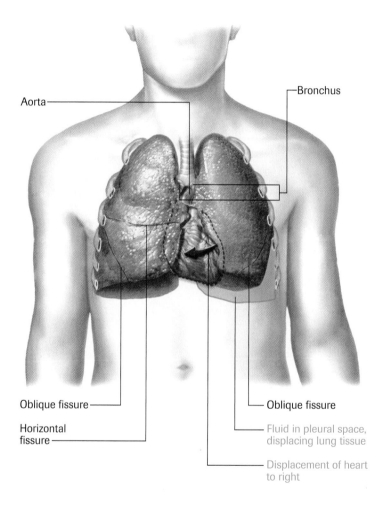

Aorta

Bronchus

Oblique fissure

Horizontal
fissure

Oblique fissure

Fluid in pleural space,
displacing lung tissue

Displacement of heart
to right

Pneumonia

- Acute infection of lung parenchyma that impairs gas exchange
- Classified by etiology, location, or type
- In bacterial pneumonia, infection triggering alveolar inflammation and edema and leading to the alveoli filling with blood and exudates and, ultimately, atelectasis
- In viral pneumonia, virus attacking bronchial epithelial cells, causing inflammation and desquamation

Causes
- Aspiration
- Bacterial or viral infection

Pathophysiologic changes

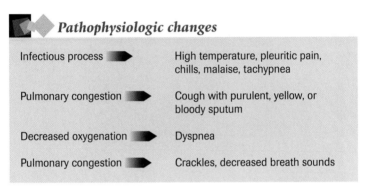

Infectious process ➡	High temperature, pleuritic pain, chills, malaise, tachypnea
Pulmonary congestion ➡	Cough with purulent, yellow, or bloody sputum
Decreased oxygenation ➡	Dyspnea
Pulmonary congestion ➡	Crackles, decreased breath sounds

TYPES OF PNEUMONIA

LOBAR PNEUMONIA   BRONCHOPNEUMONIA

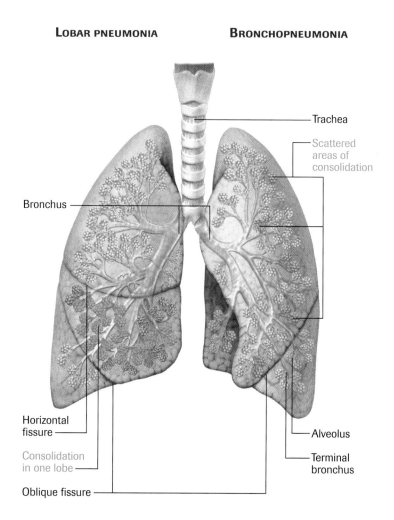

Trachea

Scattered areas of consolidation

Bronchus

Horizontal fissure

Consolidation in one lobe

Oblique fissure

Alveolus

Terminal bronchus

Pneumothorax

- Partial or complete lung collapse, caused by air in pleural cavity
- Most common types: closed, open, and tension (life-threatening)
- Spontaneous pneumothorax (type of closed pneumothorax) common among older patients with chronic pulmonary disease

Causes

- Closed pneumothorax: blunt chest trauma, air leakage from ruptured blebs, rupture resulting from barotrauma, tubercular or cancerous lesions, interstitial lung disease
- Open pneumothorax: penetrating chest injury or surgery, insertion of central venous catheter, transbronchial biopsy, thoracentesis, closed pleural biopsy
- Tension pneumothorax: penetrating chest wound treated with airtight dressing, fractured ribs, mechanical ventilation, high-level positive end-expiratory pressure, chest tube occlusion or malfunction; high pressure causes pulmonary and circulatory impairment

Pathophysiologic changes

OPEN OR CLOSED PNEUMOTHORAX

Lung collapse ➡	Sudden, sharp pain; asymmetrical chest wall movement; respiratory distress; decreased local fremitus; absent breath sounds on affected side
Hypoxia ➡	Shortness of breath, cyanosis, tachycardia
Decreased lung expansion ➡	Chest rigidity on affected side
Leakage of air into tissues ➡	Crackling beneath skin on palpation

TENSION PNEUMOTHORAX

Decreased cardiac output ➡	Hypotension, compensatory tachycardia, pallor, weak, rapid pulse
Hypoxia ➡	Tachypnea, anxiety
Increased tension ➡	Mediastinal shift
Mediastinal shift ➡	Tracheal deviation to opposite side

EFFECTS OF PNEUMOTHORAX

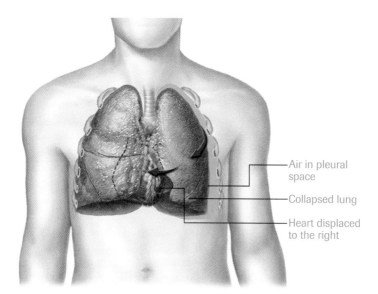

Air in pleural space

Collapsed lung

Heart displaced to the right

TENSION PNEUMOTHORAX

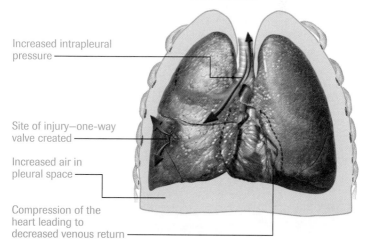

Increased intrapleural pressure

Site of injury—one-way valve created

Increased air in pleural space

Compression of the heart leading to decreased venous return

Pulmonary edema

- Accumulation of fluid in extravascular spaces of lung
- Common complication of cardiovascular disorders
- May be chronic or acute

Causes
- Acute myocardial ischemia and infarction
- Barbiturate or opiate poisoning
- Fluid overload
- Inhalation of irritating gases
- Left-sided heart failure
- Pneumonia
- Valvular heart disease

Pathophysiologic changes

EARLY STAGES

Hypoxia ➤	Dyspnea on exertion, mild tachypnea, cough, tachycardia
Decreased ability of diaphragm to expand ➤	Orthopnea
Increased pulmonary pressures ➤	Increased blood pressure
Fluid-filled lungs ➤	Dependent crackles
Decreased cardiac output and increased pulmonary vascular resistance ➤	Jugular vein distention

LATE STAGES

Hypoxia ➤	Labored, rapid respirations; increased tachycardia; cyanosis; arrhythmias
Fluid-filled lungs ➤	More diffuse crackles, cough (producing frothy, bloody sputum)
Peripheral vasoconstriction ➤	Cold, clammy skin
Decreased cardiac output, shock ➤	Diaphoresis, decreased blood pressure, thready pulse

HOW PULMONARY EDEMA DEVELOPS

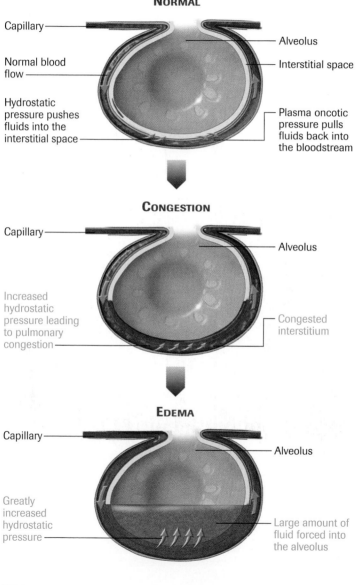

NORMAL

Capillary

Normal blood flow

Hydrostatic pressure pushes fluids into the interstitial space

Alveolus

Interstitial space

Plasma oncotic pressure pulls fluids back into the bloodstream

CONGESTION

Capillary

Increased hydrostatic pressure leading to pulmonary congestion

Alveolus

Congested interstitium

EDEMA

Capillary

Greatly increased hydrostatic pressure

Alveolus

Large amount of fluid forced into the alveolus

Pulmonary embolism

- Obstruction of pulmonary arterial bed by dislodged thrombus, heart valve growth, or foreign substance
- Most common pulmonary complication in hospitalized patients; massive embolism may be fatal

Causes
- Atrial fibrillation
- Deep vein thrombosis
- Pelvic, renal, and hepatic vein thrombosis
- Right heart thrombus
- Upper extremity thrombosis
- Valvular heart disease

Pathophysiologic changes

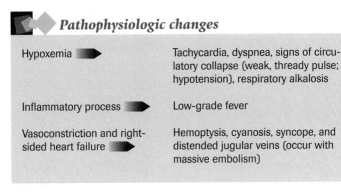

Hypoxemia ➤	Tachycardia, dyspnea, signs of circulatory collapse (weak, thready pulse; hypotension), respiratory alkalosis
Inflammatory process ➤	Low-grade fever
Vasoconstriction and right-sided heart failure ➤	Hemoptysis, cyanosis, syncope, and distended jugular veins (occur with massive embolism)

PULMONARY EMBOLI

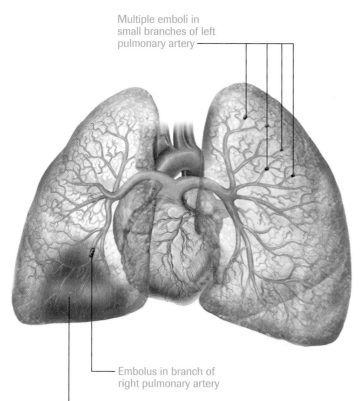

Multiple emboli in small branches of left pulmonary artery

Embolus in branch of right pulmonary artery

Infarcted area

Pulmonary hypertension

- Increase in pulmonary artery pressure (PAP) above normal (mean PAP of 25 mm HG or more) that occurs for reasons other than aging or altitude
- May be classified as primary (idiopathic) or secondary
- Primary form characterized by increased PAP and increased pulmonary vascular resistance (with no obvious cause); most common in women ages 20 to 40
- Secondary form resulting from existing cardiac or pulmonary disease

Causes
- Primary pulmonary hypertension: possible hereditary factors or altered immune mechanisms
- Secondary pulmonary hypertension: chronic obstructive pulmonary disease, diffuse interstitial pneumonia, malignant metastases, scleroderma, obesity, pulmonary embolism, vasculitis, rheumatic valvular disease, mitral stenosis

Pathophysiologic changes

Left-sided heart failure	Increasing dyspnea on exertion, difficulty breathing, shortness of breath, restlessness, agitation, decreased level of consciousness, confusion, memory loss
Diminished tissue oxygenation	Fatigue and weakness, syncope
Accumulation of lactic acid in tissues	Pain with breathing
Right ventricular failure	Ascites, jugular vein distention, peripheral edema
Hypoventilation	Possible displacement of point of maximal impulse beyond midclavicular line; decreased breath sounds; loud, tubular breath sound
Altered cardiac output	Easily palpable right ventricular lift; systolic ejection murmur; split S_2, S_3, and S_4

CHANGES IN PULMONARY HYPERTENSION

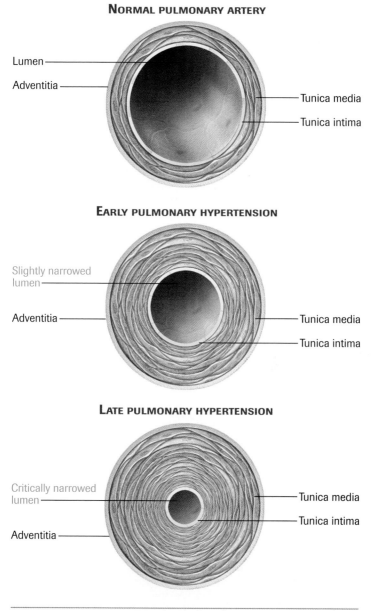

Normal pulmonary artery

Lumen

Adventitia

Tunica media

Tunica intima

Early pulmonary hypertension

Slightly narrowed lumen

Adventitia

Tunica media

Tunica intima

Late pulmonary hypertension

Critically narrowed lumen

Adventitia

Tunica media

Tunica intima

Sarcoidosis

- Multisystem, granulomatous disorder
- Evidence suggesting that disease results from exaggerated cellular immune response to a limited class of antigens
- Produces lymphadenopathy, pulmonary infiltration, and skeletal, liver, eye, or skin lesions

Cause
- Unknown

Pathophysiologic changes

Inflammatory process ➤	Granuloma formation and organ dysfunction
Alveolitis ➤	Breathlessness, cough, wheezing; substernal chest pain; pulmonary hypertension and cor pulmonale

LUNG CHANGES IN SARCOIDOSIS

NORMAL LUNGS AND ALVEOLI

GRANULOMATOUS TISSUE FORMATION

ALVEOLITIS

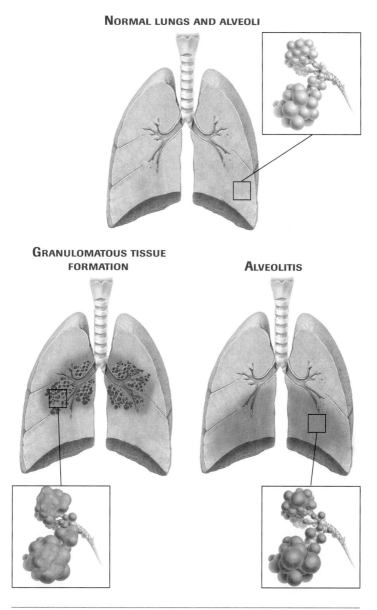

Severe acute respiratory syndrome (SARS)

- Life-threatening viral infection
- Incubation period estimated to range from 2 to 7 days
- Origin unknown, but close contact with civet cats may have transmitted a mutated form of the coronavirus to humans
- Not highly contagious when protective measures in place

Cause
- Coronavirus known as SARS-associated coronavirus
- Risk factors: contact with infected person, contact with aerosolized droplets and body secretions from infected person, and travel to endemic areas

Pathophysiologic changes

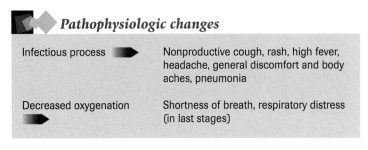

Infectious process ➡	Nonproductive cough, rash, high fever, headache, general discomfort and body aches, pneumonia
Decreased oxygenation ➡	Shortness of breath, respiratory distress (in last stages)

LUNGS AND ALVEOLI IN SARS

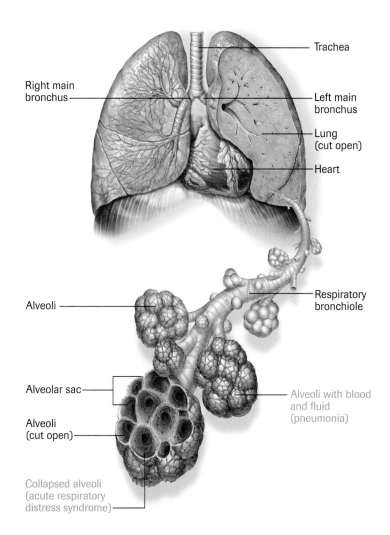

Trachea

Right main bronchus

Left main bronchus

Lung (cut open)

Heart

Alveoli

Respiratory bronchiole

Alveolar sac

Alveoli with blood and fluid (pneumonia)

Alveoli (cut open)

Collapsed alveoli (acute respiratory distress syndrome)

Tuberculosis

- Lung infection characterized by pulmonary infiltrates and formation of granulomas with caseation, fibrosis, and cavitation
- May be acute or chronic
- Excellent prognosis with proper treatment and compliance

Causes

- Exposure to *Mycobacterium tuberculosis*
- Sometimes, exposure to other strains of mycobacteria

Pathophysiologic changes

Inflammatory and immune process ➡	Fever and night sweats, malaise, weight loss, adenopathy, productive cough (lasting longer than 3 weeks), hemoptysis, pleuritic chest pain
Mycobacterium entering the lymphatic system ➡	Symptoms of airway obstruction from lymph node involvement

APPEARANCE OF TUBERCULOSIS
ON LUNG TISSUE

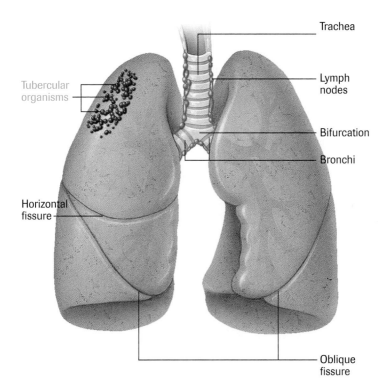

Trachea

Tubercular
organisms

Lymph
nodes

Bifurcation

Bronchi

Horizontal
fissure

Oblique
fissure

Upper respiratory tract infection

- Most common infectious disease
- Acute, usually afebrile viral infection that causes inflammation of the upper respiratory tract including the sinuses, nasopharynx, pharynx, larynx, and trachea
- Also known as the *common cold* or *acute coryza* and may lead to secondary bacterial infections

Causes
- Usually caused by rhinoviruses, coronaviruses, myxoviruses, adenoviruses, Coxsackie viruses, and echoviruses
- Viral infection of the upper respiratory passages

Pathophysiologic changes

General inflammatory reaction ➡	Fever, chills, myalgia, arthralgia, malaise, lethargy
Inflammation of the upper airway structures ➡	Pharyngitis; nasal congestion and copious nasal drainage; headache; burning, watery eyes; coryza and sneezing

COMPLICATIONS OF THE COMMON COLD

SINUSITIS

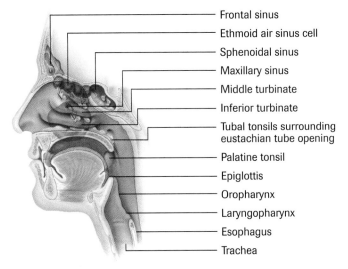

Frontal sinus
Ethmoid air sinus cell
Sphenoidal sinus
Maxillary sinus
Middle turbinate
Inferior turbinate
Tubal tonsils surrounding eustachian tube opening
Palatine tonsil
Epiglottis
Oropharynx
Laryngopharynx
Esophagus
Trachea

RHINITIS

BRONCHITIS

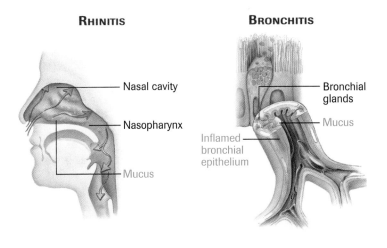

Nasal cavity
Nasopharynx
Mucus

Bronchial glands
Mucus
Inflamed bronchial epithelium

3

Neurosensory system

Acceleration-deceleration injuries

- Commonly called *whiplash*
- Cervical injury resulting from sharp hyperextension and flexion of the neck
- Damages ligaments, disks, and nerve tissue
- Symptoms commonly subsiding with treatment

Causes
- Assaults and crimes
- Falls
- Motor vehicle and other transportation accidents
- Sports-related accidents

Pathophysiologic changes

Injury to muscles in the neck ➤	Neck pain, headache, nuchal rigidity and neck muscle asymmetry
Torn, pinched, or stretched vertebral arteries ➤	Decreased blood flow to the brain
Spinal nerve injury ➤	Gait disturbances, dizziness, vomiting, rigidity or numbness in the arms

WHIPLASH INJURIES OF THE HEAD AND NECK

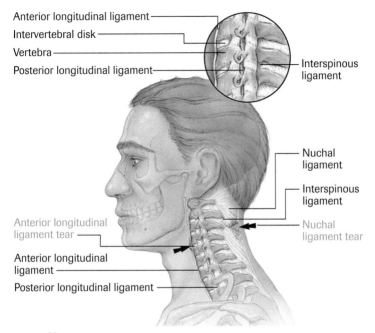

Anterior longitudinal ligament

Intervertebral disk

Vertebra

Posterior longitudinal ligament

Interspinous ligament

Nuchal ligament

Interspinous ligament

Nuchal ligament tear

Anterior longitudinal ligament tear

Anterior longitudinal ligament

Posterior longitudinal ligament

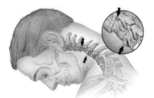

HYPERFLEXION

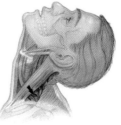

MUSCLE INJURY

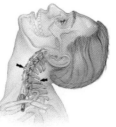

HYPEREXTENSION

Acceleration-deceleration injuries

105

Alzheimer's disease

- Degenerative disorder of the cerebral cortex that's considered primary progressive form of dementia
- Accounts for more than one-half of all cases of dementia
- Carries a poor prognosis

Causes
- Unknown
- Environmental factors: exposure to aluminum or manganese; repeated head trauma
- Neurochemical factors: deficiencies in neurotransmitters acetylcholine, norepinephrine, serotonin, and somatostatin

Pathophysiologic changes

Neurotransmitter metabolism defect ➤	Initial stage: Gradual loss of recent and remote memory, disorientation (time, date), flattening of affect and personality
Neurotransmitter metabolism deficits or structural loss of brain tissue ➤	Progressive stages: Impaired cognition; inability to concentrate; difficulty with abstraction and judgment; inability to perform activities of daily living; restlessness and agitation; personality changes; nocturnal awakening and wandering; severe deterioration in memory, language, and motor function; loss of coordination; inability to write or speak; loss of eye contact; acute confusion, agitation, compulsive behavior, fearfulness; disorientation and emotional lability; urinary and fecal incontinence

TISSUE CHANGES IN ALZHEIMER'S DISEASE

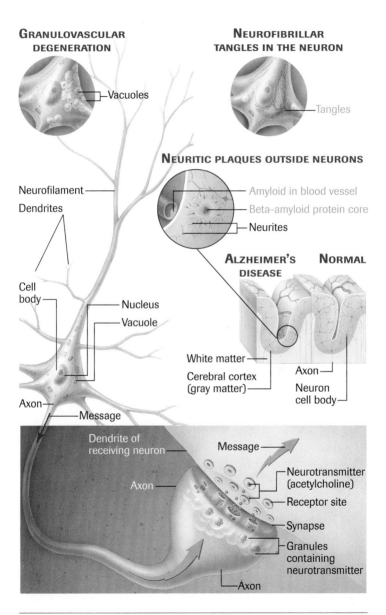

GRANULOVASCULAR DEGENERATION

Vacuoles

NEUROFIBRILLAR TANGLES IN THE NEURON

Tangles

NEURITIC PLAQUES OUTSIDE NEURONS

Amyloid in blood vessel

Beta-amyloid protein core

Neurites

Neurofilament

Dendrites

ALZHEIMER'S DISEASE

NORMAL

Cell body

Nucleus

Vacuole

White matter

Cerebral cortex (gray matter)

Axon

Neuron cell body

Axon

Message

Dendrite of receiving neuron

Message

Axon

Neurotransmitter (acetylcholine)

Receptor site

Synapse

Granules containing neurotransmitter

Axon

Amyotrophic
lateral sclerosis

- Chronic, progressively debilitating disease, commonly called *ALS* or *Lou Gehrig's disease*
- Most common form of motor neuron disease causing muscular atrophy
- Onset usually occurs between ages 40 and 60
- Affects men twice as commonly as women

Causes

- Unknown; 5% to 10% of cases have genetic component
- Possible contributing mechanisms: autoimmune disorder, nutritional deficiency related to disturbance in enzyme metabolism, slow-acting virus, unknown mechanism that causes buildup of excess glutamine in cerebrospinal fluid

Pathophysiologic changes

Degeneration of upper and lower motor neurons ➡	Fasciculations accompanied by spasticity, atrophy, hyperreflexia and weakness (especially in muscles of forearms and hands), muscle atrophy
	Degeneration of cranial nerves V, IX, X, and XII
	Impaired speech, difficulty chewing and swallowing, choking, and excessive drooling
Brain stem involvement ➡	Difficulty breathing
Progressive bulbar palsy ➡	Emotional lability

MOTOR NEURON CHANGES IN ALS

NORMAL NERVE CELL AND MUSCLE

ALS-AFFECTED NERVE CELL AND MUSCLE

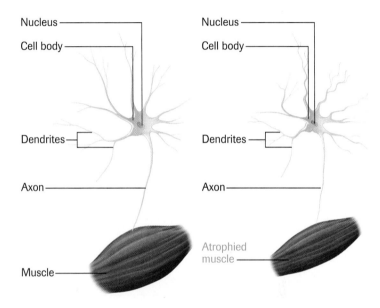

Nucleus

Cell body

Dendrites

Axon

Muscle

Nucleus

Cell body

Dendrites

Axon

Atrophied muscle

Arteriovenous malformation

- Tangled masses of thin-walled, dilated vessels between arteries and veins that aren't connected by capillaries
- Commonly found in the posterior portion of the cerebral hemisphere
- Leading to mixing of oxygenated and unoxygenated blood and leading to inadequate cerebral perfusion
- Range in size from a few millimeters to large malformations extending from the cerebral cortex to the ventricles
- Usually more than one exists

Causes
- Acquired; trauma such as penetrating injuries
- Congenital; hereditary defect

Pathophysiologic changes

Intracranial hemorrhage ➡	Severe headache, seizures, confusion, lethargy, and meningeal irritation
Compression of surrounding tissues by engorged vessels ➡	Seizures
Turbulent blood flow ➡	Systolic bruit over carotid artery, mastoid process, or orbit
Diminished cerebral perfusion ➡	Focal neurologic deficits
Extension of arteriovenous malformation into the ventricular lining ➡	Hydrocephalus

ARTERIOVENOUS MALFORMATION

CEREBRAL CORTEX—SAGITTAL SECTION

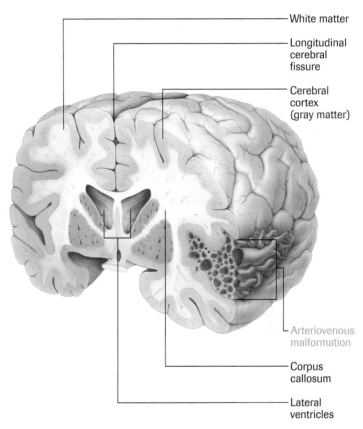

White matter

Longitudinal cerebral fissure

Cerebral cortex (gray matter)

Arteriovenous malformation

Corpus callosum

Lateral ventricles

Brain tumors

- Abnormal growths in the brain, cerebral vasculature, or meninges
- Most common types: gliomas, meningiomas, and pituitary adenomas
- Usually referred to as benign or malignant
- Malignant brain tumors: grow and multiply rapidly
- Benign tumors: possibly neurologically devastating depending on the size and location

Causes
- Unknown in most cases
- Genetic loss or mutation
- Prior cranial radiation exposure

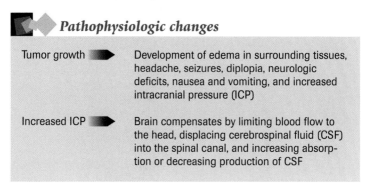

Pathophysiologic changes

Tumor growth ➤	Development of edema in surrounding tissues, headache, seizures, diplopia, neurologic deficits, nausea and vomiting, and increased intracranial pressure (ICP)
Increased ICP ➤	Brain compensates by limiting blood flow to the head, displacing cerebrospinal fluid (CSF) into the spinal canal, and increasing absorption or decreasing production of CSF

PRIMARY BRAIN TUMOR

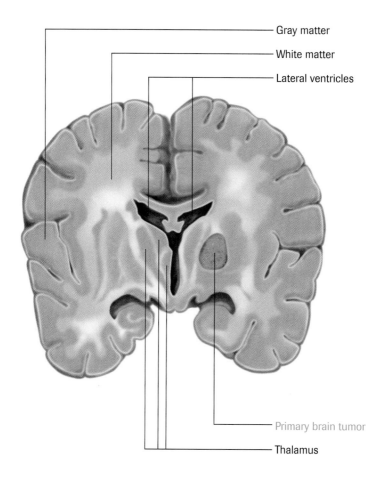

Gray matter

White matter

Lateral ventricles

Primary brain tumor

Thalamus

Cataract

- Gradually developing opacity of the lens or lens capsule of the eye
- Light shining through the cornea becoming blocked by opacity causing hazy image
- Usually developing bilaterally, but each progressing independently unless it's traumatic (develop unilaterally) or congenital (remain stationary)
- Surgery improving vision in 95% of affected people

Causes
- Aging
- Atopic dermatitis
- Drugs that are toxic to the lens
- Exposure to radiation
- Genetic abnormalities
- Glaucoma, retinal disorders, uveitis
- Infection
- Maternal malnutrition
- Metabolic diseases
- Myotonic dystrophy
- Trauma

Pathophysiologic changes

Lens opacity ➡	Gradual painless blurring and loss of vision; milky white pupil
Ineffective reflection of light ➡	Blinding glare from headlight or bright lights at night; better vision in dim light
Reduced visual clarity ➡	Poor reading vision

UNDERSTANDING CATARACT

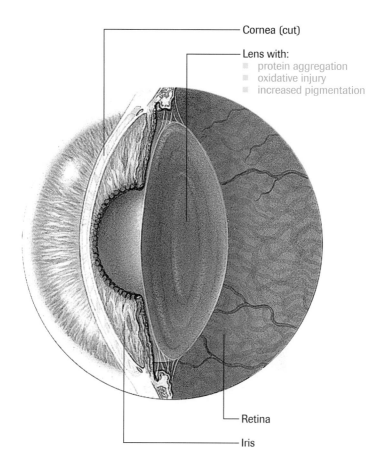

Cornea (cut)

Lens with:
- protein aggregation
- oxidative injury
- increased pigmentation

Retina

Iris

Cerebral aneurysm

- Weakness in wall of a cerebral artery, leading to localized dilation
- Usually arises at arterial junction in Circle of Willis
- Rupture common, resulting in subarachnoid hemorrhage
- Rupture severity graded according to signs and symptoms

Causes

- Combination of congenital defect and degenerative process
- Congenital defect
- Degenerative process
- Traumatic injury

Pathophysiologic changes

PREMONITORY STAGE

Oozing of blood into subarachnoid space ▶	Headache, nausea, vomiting; nuchal rigidity; stiff back and legs

RUPTURE STAGE

Increased pressure from bleeding into enclosed space ▶	Severe headache; nausea and projectile vomiting; altered level of consciousness, including coma
Bleeding into meninges ▶	Meningeal irritation including nuchal rigidity, back and leg pain, fever, restlessness, irritability, occasional seizures, photophobia, blurred vision
Bleeding into brain tissues ▶	Hemiparesis, dysphagia, and vision deficits
Compression on oculomotor nerve if the aneurysm is near the internal carotid artery ▶	Diplopia, ptosis, dilated pupil, inability to rotate the eye

UNDERSTANDING CEREBRAL ANEURYSM

CIRCLE OF WILLIS

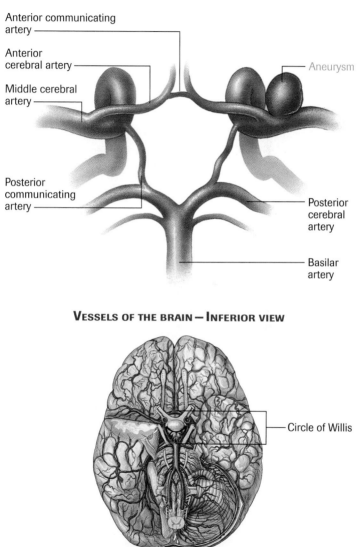

Anterior communicating artery

Anterior cerebral artery

Middle cerebral artery

Aneurysm

Posterior communicating artery

Posterior cerebral artery

Basilar artery

VESSELS OF THE BRAIN — INFERIOR VIEW

Circle of Willis

Cleft lip and cleft palate

- Occurs separately or in combination
- Originates in the second month of pregnancy
- Cleft lip: occurs unilaterally, bilaterally, or in the midline; may involve only the lip or extend into the upper jaw or nasal cavity

Causes
- Chromosomal abnormality (trisomy 13)
- Combination of environmental and genetic factors
- Exposure to teratogens during fetal development

Pathophysiologic changes

Imperfect fusion of the front and sides of the face and the palatine shelves ➡	Notch in the upper lip, complete cleft from the lip edge through the floor of the nostril, or partial or complete cleft of the soft and hard palate
Incomplete fusion of the palate or abnormality of the lip ➡	Feeding difficulties and malnutrition
Middle ear damage or recurrent ear infections ➡	Hearing impairment
Ineffective speech patterns continue after surgical correction ➡	Permanent speech impediment

VARIATIONS OF CLEFT DEFORMITY

CLEFT LIP

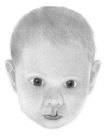

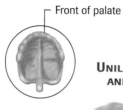

Front of palate

UNILATERAL CLEFT LIP AND CLEFT PALATE

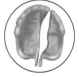

BILATERAL CLEFT LIP AND CLEFT PALATE

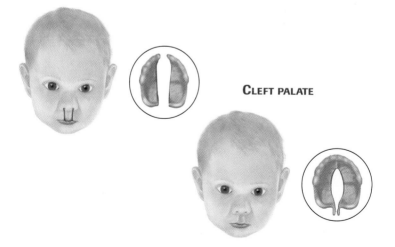

CLEFT PALATE

Depression

- Chronic and recurrent mood disorder
- Symptoms interfering with everyday life for an extended period
- Reported to be underdiagnosed and inadequately treated
- Includes dysthymia, major depression, premenstrual dysphoric disorder, postpartum depression, and seasonal affective disorder

Causes
- Genetic predisposition
- Imbalance of neurotransmitters
- Several contributing factors: death of family member or friend, drug and alcohol abuse, nutritional deficiencies, prolonged illness or pain, sleep problems, social isolation, and stress

Pathophysiologic changes

Inadequate levels of serotonin or norepinephrine ➡	Sad, anxious or "empty" mood; hopelessness and pessimism; feelings of guilt, worthlessness, and helplessness; loss of interest in activities or hobbies; loss of energy; unexplained pain; GI symptoms; headache; insomnia; dizziness; palpitations; heartburn; numbness; loss of appetite; premenstrual syndrome

UNDERSTANDING DEPRESSION

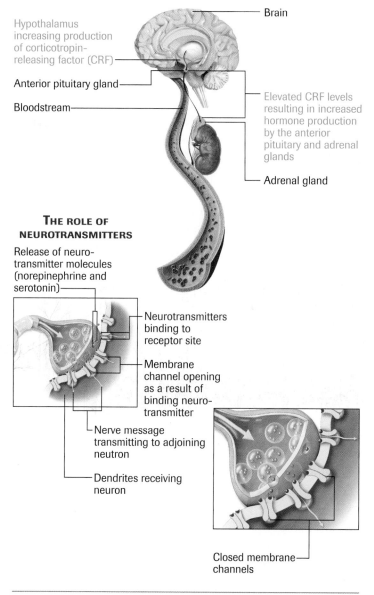

Brain

Hypothalamus increasing production of corticotropin-releasing factor (CRF)

Anterior pituitary gland

Bloodstream

Elevated CRF levels resulting in increased hormone production by the anterior pituitary and adrenal glands

Adrenal gland

THE ROLE OF NEUROTRANSMITTERS

Release of neuro-transmitter molecules (norepinephrine and serotonin)

Neurotransmitters binding to receptor site

Membrane channel opening as a result of binding neuro-transmitter

Nerve message transmitting to adjoining neutron

Dendrites receiving neuron

Closed membrane channels

Epilepsy

- Condition of the brain characterized by susceptibility to recurrent seizures
- Primary epilepsy: idiopathic and not related to structural changes in the brain
- Secondary epilepsy: characterized by structural changes in the brain

Causes

- Anoxia
- Birth trauma
- Brain tumors
- Head injury or trauma
- Idiopathic
- Infectious diseases of the brain
- Ingestion of toxins
- Inherited disorders
- Metabolic disorders
- Perinatal infection
- Stroke

Pathophysiologic changes

Abnormal electrical discharge of neurons in the brain ➥	Tonic stiffening followed by clonic muscular contractions; tongue biting; incontinence; blank stare; purposeless motor activities; change in level of awareness; loss of postural tone; jerking and twitching
Brain's increased demand for oxygen ➥	Hypoxia, labored breathing, cyanosis, apnea, and brain damage

TYPES OF SEIZURES

GENERALIZED SEIZURE

COMPLEX-PARTIAL SEIZURE

SIMPLE-PARTIAL SEIZURE

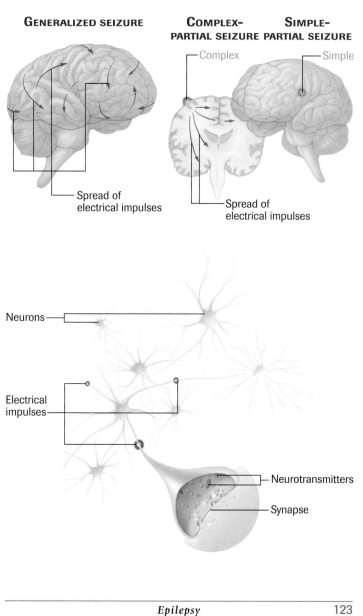

Complex

Simple

Spread of
electrical impulses

Spread of
electrical impulses

Neurons

Electrical
impulses

Neurotransmitters

Synapse

Glaucoma

- Characterized by abnormally high intraocular pressure
- Leads to damage of the optic nerve and other intraocular structures
- Untreated, leads to vision loss and blindness
- Chronic open-angle glaucoma: bilateral with a slow, insidious onset
- Acute angle-closure glaucoma: rapid onset; medical emergency

Causes

CHRONIC OPEN-ANGLE GLAUCOMA

- Aging
- Diabetes mellitus
- Genetics
- Hypertension
- Myopia

ACUTE ANGLE-CLOSURE GLAUCOMA

- Drug-induced
- Excitement or stress leading to hypertension

SECONDARY GLAUCOMA

- Diabetes
- Infections
- Steroids
- Surgery
- Trauma
- Uveitis

Pathophysiologic changes

Increased intraocular pressure ➤	Eye pain and pressure, nausea and vomiting, photophobia
Corneal edema ➤	Halos around lights
Compression of rods and nerve fibers ➤	Loss of vision, decreased acuity and blurring

OPTIC DISK CHANGES IN GLAUCOMA

NORMAL OPTIC DISK

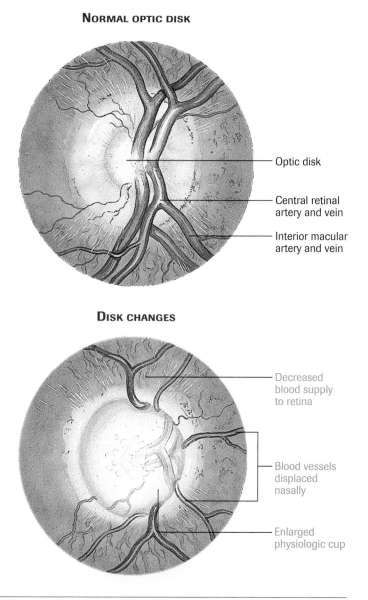

Optic disk

Central retinal
artery and vein

Interior macular
artery and vein

DISK CHANGES

Decreased
blood supply
to retina

Blood vessels
displaced
nasally

Enlarged
physiologic cup

Guillain-Barré syndrome

- Rapidly progressive and potentially fatal motor neuropathy
- Symptoms peaking within 7 days to 4 weeks of onset
- Permanent weakness or disability occurring in 10% to 25% of cases

Causes
- Unknown
- In many cases, viral infection that produces an immune response
- Other precipitating factors: certain drugs, collagen vascular disease, hematologic malignancies, hyperthyroidism, immunizations, pregnancy, sarcoidosis, surgery, and transplants

Pathophysiologic changes

Impaired anterior nerve root transmission ▶	Symmetrical muscle weakness starting in the legs and ascending to the arms and facial nerves (ascending) or muscle weakness in the arms or arms and legs simultaneously
Impaired dorsal nerve root transmission ▶	Paresthesia
Interruption of the reflex arc ▶	Hypotonia and areflexia
Cranial nerve involvement ▶	Diplegia, ocular paralysis, dysphagia, and dysarthria

PERIPHERAL NERVE DEMYELINATION

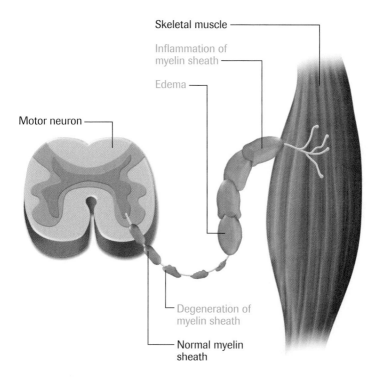

Skeletal muscle

Inflammation of
myelin sheath

Edema

Motor neuron

Degeneration of
myelin sheath

Normal myelin
sheath

Hearing loss

- Inability to perceive the normal range of sounds audible to individuals with normal hearing
- Results from mechanical or nervous impediment to the transmission of sound waves
- Types: congenital hearing loss, sudden deafness, noise-induced hearing loss, and presbycusis

Causes

- Bacterial or viral infection
- Congenital abnormalities
- Exposure to loud noises
- Inherited disorder
- Loss of hair cells in the organ of Corti
- Ototoxic drugs
- Prolonged fetal anoxia or trauma

Pathophysiologic changes

Dysfunction of conduction and sensorineural transmission ➡	Deficient response to auditory stimuli; impaired speech development; loss of perception of specific frequencies; tinnitus; and inability to understand the spoken word

CAUSES OF CONDUCTIVE HEARING LOSS

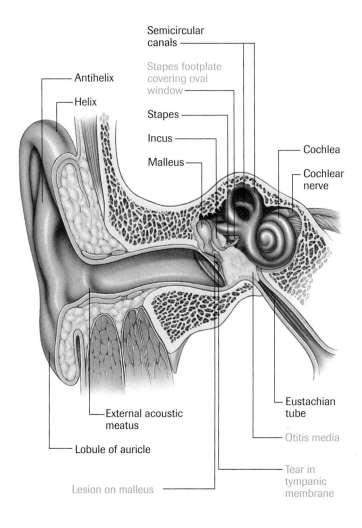

Semicircular canals

Stapes footplate covering oval window

Stapes

Incus

Malleus

Antihelix

Helix

Cochlea

Cochlear nerve

External acoustic meatus

Lobule of auricle

Lesion on malleus

Eustachian tube

Otitis media

Tear in tympanic membrane

Herniated
intervertebral disk

- Protrusion of part of gelatinous center of intervertebral disk through tear in posterior rim of outer ring
- Usually occurring in adults older than age 45
- About 90% occurring in the lumbar and lumbosacral regions

Causes
- Degenerative disk disease
- Severe strain or trauma

Pathophysiologic changes

Compression of nerve roots supplying buttocks, legs, and feet ➤	Severe lower back pain and sciatic pain
Pressure and irritation of sciatic nerve root ➤	Muscle spasms
Inactivity ➤	Weakness and atrophy of leg muscles in later stages

HERNIATION AND PAIN IN DISK INJURY

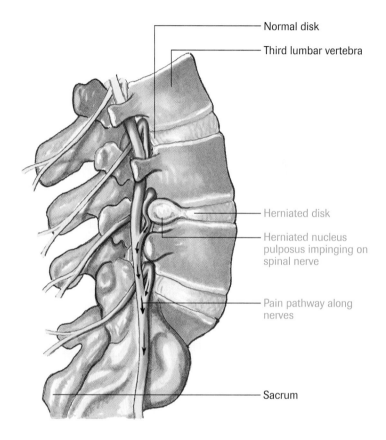

Normal disk

Third lumbar vertebra

Herniated disk

Herniated nucleus pulposus impinging on spinal nerve

Pain pathway along nerves

Sacrum

Hydrocephalus

- Excessive accumulation of cerebrospinal fluid (CSF) in the brain
- Results in increased intracranial pressure (ICP) and enlargement of the ventricular system
- Congenital or acquired and communicating or non-communicating (obstructive)

Causes
- Complication of premature birth
- Developmental disorders
- Genetic inheritance
- Possible associations: head injury, subarachnoid hemorrhage, tumors

Pathophysiologic changes

Increased CSF volume ➤	Enlargement of the head disproportionate to the infant's growth, distended scalp veins, underdeveloped neck muscles, ataxia, and thin, shiny, fragile-looking scalp skin
Increased ICP ➤	Depressed orbital roof with downward displacement of the eyes, prominent sclera, impaired intellect, projectile vomiting, decreased level of consciousness, and skull widening

UNDERSTANDING HYDROCEPHALUS

NORMAL BRAIN – LATERAL VIEW

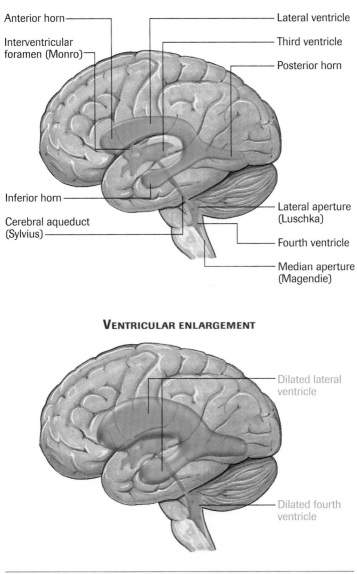

Anterior horn

Interventricular foramen (Monro)

Inferior horn

Cerebral aqueduct (Sylvius)

Lateral ventricle

Third ventricle

Posterior horn

Lateral aperture (Luschka)

Fourth ventricle

Median aperture (Magendie)

VENTRICULAR ENLARGEMENT

Dilated lateral ventricle

Dilated fourth ventricle

Intracranial hemorrhage

- Accumulation of blood in the skull
- Results from epidural, intracerebral, or subdural hematoma
- Generally produces some degree of brain injury

Causes
- Anticoagulation therapy
- Bleeding disorders
- Epidural, intracerebral, or subdural hematoma
- Head trauma
- Hypertension
- Ruptured aneurysm
- Skull fracture
- Stroke

Pathophysiologic changes

Increased pressure from bleeding into enclosed space ➤	Severe headache, nausea and projectile vomiting, and altered level of consciousness, including coma
Bleeding into meninges ➤	Meningeal irritation including nuchal rigidity, back and leg pain, fever, restlessness, irritability, occasional seizures, photophobia, blurred vision
Bleeding into brain tissues ➤	Hemiparesis, dysphagia, and vision deficits
Compression on oculomotor nerve (if aneurysm is near the internal carotid artery) ➤	Diplopia, ptosis, dilated pupil, inability to rotate the eye

COMMON SITES OF INTRACRANIAL HEMORRHAGE

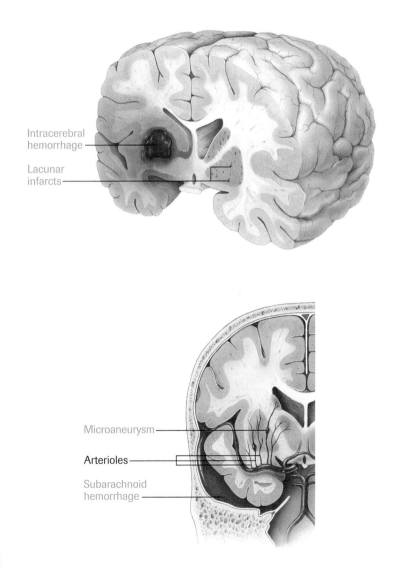

Intracerebral hemorrhage

Lacunar infarcts

Microaneurysm

Arterioles

Subarachnoid hemorrhage

Laryngeal cancer

- Malignant cells in the tissue of the larynx (voice box)
- Most common form: squamous cell carcinoma
- Classified according to location: supraglottis, glottis, or subglottis

Causes
- Unknown
- Risk factors: alcoholism, familial tendency, history of gastroesophageal reflux disease, inhalation of noxious fumes, and smoking

Pathophysiologic changes

Tumor formation in the larynx ➤	Hoarseness that persists for longer than 3 weeks, lump in the throat, pain or burning in the throat when drinking citrus juice or hot liquids, dysphagia, pain radiating to the ear, and enlarged cervical lymph nodes
Partial airway obstruction ➤	Dyspnea, lump in the throat, cough

UNDERSTANDING LARYNGEAL CANCER

MIRROR VIEW

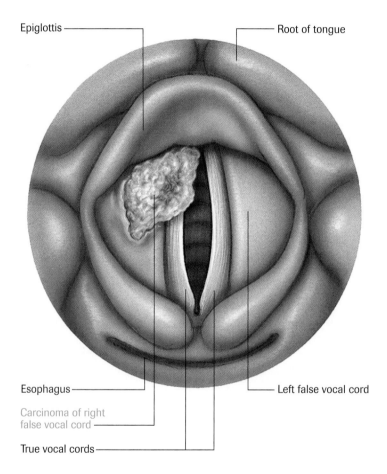

Epiglottis

Root of tongue

Esophagus

Left false vocal cord

Carcinoma of right
false vocal cord

True vocal cords

Lyme disease

- Multisystem disorder caused by *Borrelia burgdorferi* (spirochete transmitted through tick bite)
- Primarily occurs in areas inhabited by small deer tick (*Ixodes dammini*)
- Typically manifests in three stages: Early localized stage (distinctive rash accompanied by flulike symptoms); early disseminated stage (neurologic and cardiac abnormalities); late stage (arthritis, chronic neurologic problems)

Causes
- Infestation of spirochete *B. burgdorferi* resulting from tick bite

Pathophysiologic changes

EARLY LOCALIZED STAGE

Local infection of *B. burgdorferi* spirochete ➤	Distinctive red rash that appears as target or bull's eye (commonly at the site of the tick bite), flulike symptoms (fever, chills, myalgias, headache, malaise), regional lymphadenopathy

EARLY DISSEMINATED STAGE

Dissemination of spirochetes into bloodstream ➤	Neurologic (peripheral and cranial neuropathy), cardiac (carditis, conduction disturbances), and eye abnormalities (conjunctivitis)

LATE STAGE

Presence of organisms in synovium ➤	Inflammation, joint swelling, arthritis

LYME DISEASE ORGANISM AND LESION

MICROSCOPIC VIEW OF *B. BURGDORFERI*

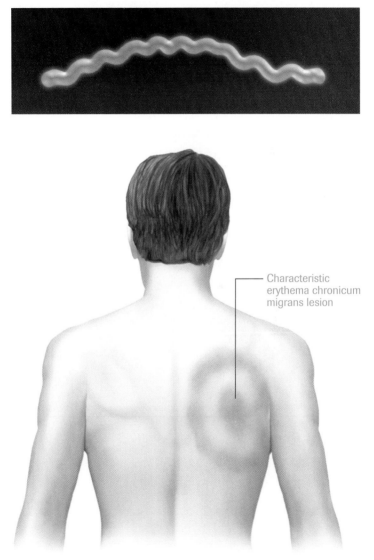

Characteristic
erythema chronicum
migrans lesion

Macular degeneration

- Atrophy or degeneration of the macular disk
- Most common cause of legal blindness in adults
- Commonly affects both eyes
- A cause of irreversible and unpreventable loss of central vision in elderly people

Causes

- Aging
- Infection
- Inflammation
- Poor nutrition
- Trauma

Pathophysiologic changes

Retinal pigment epithelium detachment and atrophy ➤	Blurry vision, vision loss
Changes in central vision ➤	Blank spot in the center of a page when reading
Relocation of retinal receptors ➤	Distorted appearance of straight lines

RETINAL CHANGES IN
MACULAR DEGENERATION

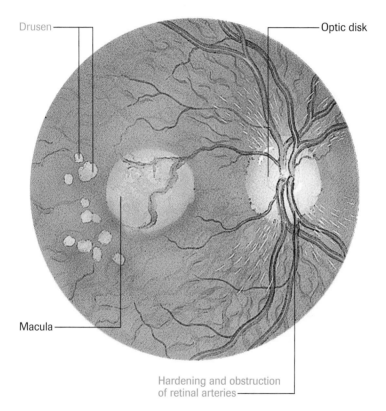

Drusen

Optic disk

Macula

Hardening and obstruction
of retinal arteries

Ménière's disease

- Labyrinthine dysfunction that causes vertigo, sensorimotor hearing loss, and tinnitus
- Usually involves one ear
- After multiple attacks, causes incapacitating tinnitus and hearing loss

Causes

- Unknown
- Possible associations: autonomic nervous system dysfunction, family history, head trauma, immune disorder, middle ear infection, migraine headaches, premenstrual edema

Pathophysiologic changes

Increased fluid in the labyrinth of the ear ▶	Severe spinning, whirling vertigo lasting 10 minutes to several hours
Altered firing of sensory auditory neurons ▶	Tinnitus
Sensorineural loss ▶	Hearing impairment
Autonomic dysfunction ▶	Nausea, vomiting, sweating and pallor
Change in sensitivity of pressure receptors ▶	Feeling of fullness or blockage in the ear
Altered impulses reaching the brain ▶	Nystagmus

UNDERSTANDING MÉNIÈRE'S DISEASE

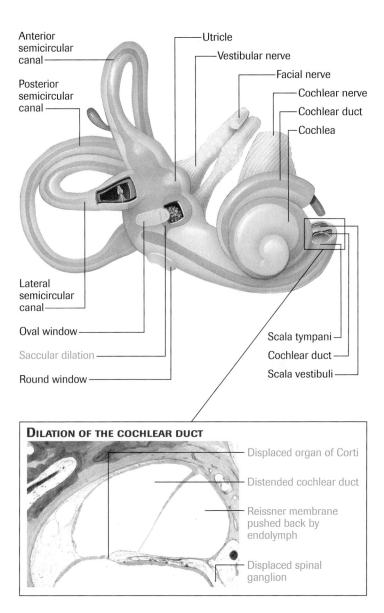

Anterior semicircular canal

Posterior semicircular canal

Lateral semicircular canal

Oval window

Saccular dilation

Round window

Utricle

Vestibular nerve

Facial nerve

Cochlear nerve

Cochlear duct

Cochlea

Scala tympani

Cochlear duct

Scala vestibuli

DILATION OF THE COCHLEAR DUCT

Displaced organ of Corti

Distended cochlear duct

Reissner membrane pushed back by endolymph

Displaced spinal ganglion

Meningitis

- Inflammation of brain and spinal cord meninges, usually resulting from bacterial infection
- May involve inflammation of all three meningeal membranes: dura mater, arachnoid, and pia mater
- Complications rare if diagnosed and treated promptly

Causes
- Complication of bacterial infection
- In some cases no causative organism
- Invasive procedures or trauma
- Virus

Pathophysiologic changes

Infection and inflammation	Fever, chills, and malaise
Increased intracranial pressure (ICP)	Headache, vomiting, and papilledema
Meningeal irritation	Nuchal rigidity, positive Brudzinski's and Kernig's signs, exaggerated and symmetrical deep tendon reflexes, opisthotonos
Irritation of nerves of autonomic nervous system	Sinus arrhythmias
Increasing ICP	Irritability, delirium, deep stupor, coma
Cranial nerve irritation	Photophobia, diplopia, and other vision problems

MENINGES AND CEREBROSPINAL FLUID FLOW

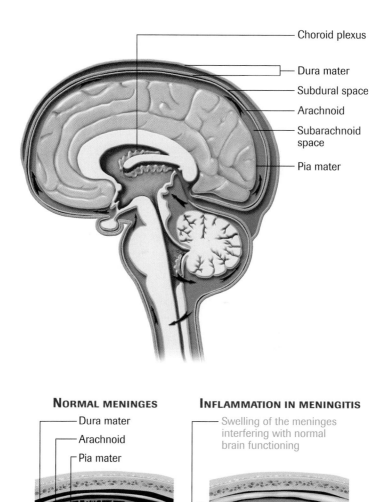

Choroid plexus

Dura mater

Subdural space

Arachnoid

Subarachnoid space

Pia mater

NORMAL MENINGES

Dura mater

Arachnoid

Pia mater

INFLAMMATION IN MENINGITIS

Swelling of the meninges interfering with normal brain functioning

Migraine headache

- Throbbing, vascular headache usually appearing in childhood and commonly recurring throughout adulthood
- May be classified according to presence of aura: common migraine (no aura); classic migraine (aura)
- More common in women; strong familial incidence

Causes
- Unknown
- Contributing triggering factors: caffeine intake, change in routine, emotional stress or fatigue, environmental stimuli, missed meals
- Triggering mechanism: neuronal dysfunction, possibly of trigeminal nerve pathway

Pathophysiologic changes

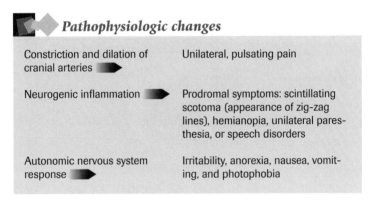

Constriction and dilation of cranial arteries ➡	Unilateral, pulsating pain
Neurogenic inflammation ➡	Prodromal symptoms: scintillating scotoma (appearance of zig-zag lines), hemianopia, unilateral paresthesia, or speech disorders
Autonomic nervous system response ➡	Irritability, anorexia, nausea, vomiting, and photophobia

VASCULAR CHANGES IN HEADACHE

NORMAL

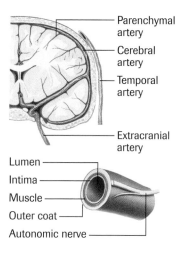

Parenchymal artery

Cerebral artery

Temporal artery

Extracranial artery

Lumen
Intima
Muscle
Outer coat
Autonomic nerve

VASOCONSTRICTION (AURA) PHASE

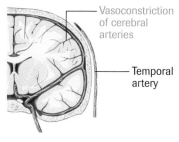

Vasoconstriction of cerebral arteries

Temporal artery

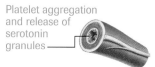

Platelet aggregation and release of serotonin granules

PARENCHYMAL ARTERY DILATION

Parenchymal artery dilation

Cerebral artery

Temporal artery

Arteriovenous shunts

Sensitive arterioles

Small artery distention

Pain impulse

VASODILATION (HEADACHE) PHASE

Cerebral artery

Vasodilation

Temporal artery

Perivascular inflammation

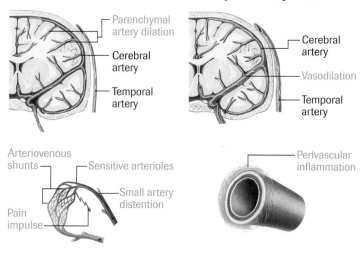

Multiple sclerosis

- Chronic disease characterized by progressive demyelination of white matter of brain and spinal cord, with periods of exacerbation and remission
- Major cause of chronic disability in young adults
- More common among women and in urban populations and upper socioeconomic groups

Causes
- Unknown
- Possible causes: environmental or genetic factors, slow-acting or latent viral infection that triggers autoimmune response
- Conditions that may precede onset or exacerbations: acute respiratory infections, emotional stress, fatigue, pregnancy

Pathophysiologic changes

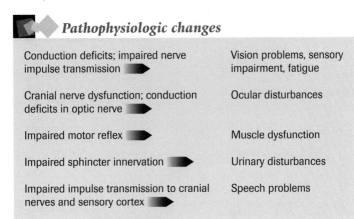

Conduction deficits; impaired nerve impulse transmission ➤	Vision problems, sensory impairment, fatigue
Cranial nerve dysfunction; conduction deficits in optic nerve ➤	Ocular disturbances
Impaired motor reflex ➤	Muscle dysfunction
Impaired sphincter innervation ➤	Urinary disturbances
Impaired impulse transmission to cranial nerves and sensory cortex ➤	Speech problems

MYELIN DESTRUCTION IN
MULTIPLE SCLEROSIS

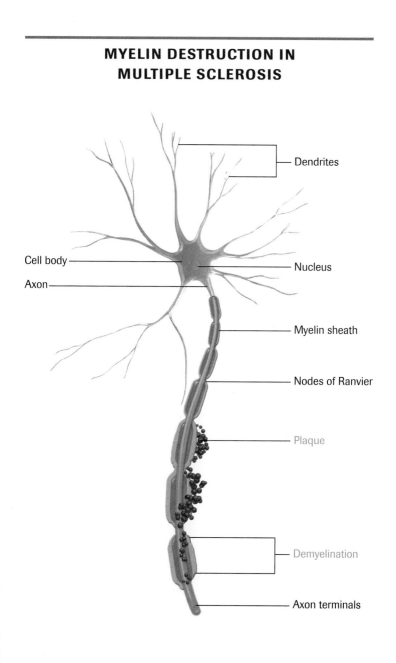

Dendrites

Cell body

Nucleus

Axon

Myelin sheath

Nodes of Ranvier

Plaque

Demyelination

Axon terminals

Myasthenia gravis

- Causes sporadic but progressive weakness and abnormal fatigability of striated muscles
- Typically affects muscles innervated by cranial nerves, but may affect any muscle group
- Symptoms exacerbated by exercise and repeated movement

Causes
- Unknown
- May result from autoimmune response, inadequate muscle fiber response to acetylcholine, or ineffective acetylcholine release

Pathophysiologic changes

Impaired neuromuscular transmission to cranial nerves supplying eye muscles →	Weak eye closure, ptosis, diplopia
Impaired neuromuscular transmission to skeletal muscles →	Skeletal muscle weakness and fatigue; muscle weakness increases throughout day and deceases with rest; paralysis in late stages; muscle weakness more intense during menses and after stress, prolonged exposure to sunlight or cold, and infections
Impaired transmission of cranial nerves innervating facial muscles →	Blank, expressionless facial appearance; nasal vocal tones
Cranial nerve involvement →	Nasal regurgitation of fluids, difficulty chewing and swallowing
Weakened facial and extraocular muscles →	Drooping eyelids
Impaired neuromuscular transmission to the diaphragm →	Difficulty breathing, predisposition to pneumonia and other respiratory tract infections

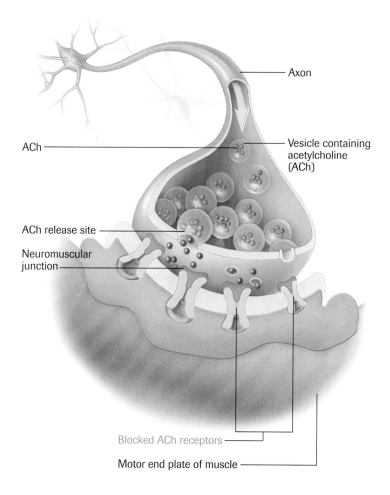

Axon

ACh

Vesicle containing acetylcholine (ACh)

ACh release site

Neuromuscular junction

Blocked ACh receptors

Motor end plate of muscle

Otitis media

- Inflammation of the middle ear
- Common in children; incidence rises during winter months
- In chronic cases, possible structural and functional ear damage and hearing loss

Causes
- Bacterial infection
- Barotrauma
- Edema from allergic rhinitis or chronic sinus infection
- Mechanical obstruction
- Obstruction of the eustachian tube
- Tuberculosis

Pathophysiologic changes

Pressure behind the tympanic membrane ➤	Severe, deep throbbing pain; bulging tympanic membrane; sensation of ear fullness; conductive hearing loss; tinnitus; dizziness; nausea and vomiting
Tympanic membrane rupture ➤	Bulging, erythematous tympanic membrane; purulent drainage in the ear canal
Infection and inflammation ➤	Fever, malaise

CLASSIFICATION OF OTITIS MEDIA

ACUTE OTITIS MEDIA

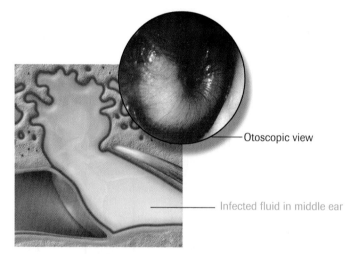

Otoscopic view

Infected fluid in middle ear

OTITIS MEDIA WITH EFFUSION

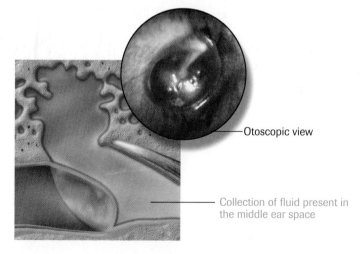

Otoscopic view

Collection of fluid present in the middle ear space

Parkinson's disease

- Degenerative disease
- Produces progressive muscle rigidity, akinesia, and involuntary tremor

Causes
- Unknown
- Possibly caused by dopamine deficiency or exposure to toxins

Pathophysiologic changes

Loss of inhibitory dopamine activity at synapse ➤	Muscle rigidity, akinesia, insidious "pill-rolling" tremor; tremor increasing during stress or anxiety and decreasing with purposeful movement and sleep
Depletion of dopamine ➤	Muscle rigidity with resistance to passive muscle stretching; may be uniform or jerky; high-pitched, monotone voice; mask-like facial expression; loss of postural tone
Impaired regulation of motor function ➤	Drooling
Autonomic dysfunction ➤	Dysarthria, dysphagia, excessive sweating, decreased motility of GI and genitourinary smooth muscle
Impaired vascular smooth muscle response ➤	Orthostatic hypotension
Inappropriate androgen production ➤	Oily skin

NEUROTRANSMITTER ACTION IN PARKINSON'S DISEASE

BRAIN – CORONAL SECTION

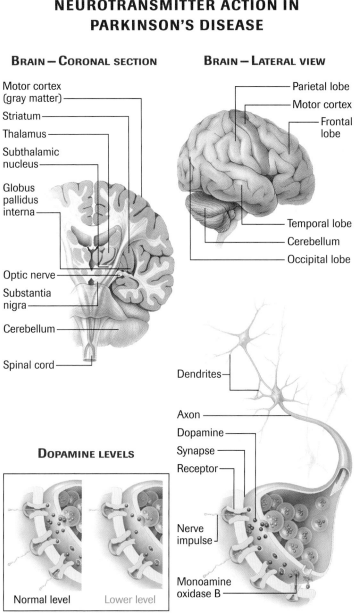

Motor cortex
(gray matter)

Striatum

Thalamus

Subthalamic
nucleus

Globus
pallidus
interna

Optic nerve

Substantia
nigra

Cerebellum

Spinal cord

BRAIN – LATERAL VIEW

Parietal lobe

Motor cortex

Frontal
lobe

Temporal lobe

Cerebellum

Occipital lobe

Dendrites

Axon

Dopamine

Synapse

Receptor

Nerve
impulse

Monoamine
oxidase B

DOPAMINE LEVELS

Normal level   Lower level

Spina bifida

- Congenital malformations that produce defects of the spine or skull
- Results from failure of neural tube closure
- Categorized into two types: spina bifida occulta and spina bifida cystica
- Two major forms of spina bifida cystica: meningocele and myelomeningocele

Causes

- Combination of environmental and genetic factors
- Exposure to teratogen
- Lack of dietary folic acid intake at time of conception
- Part of multiple malformation syndrome

Pathophysiologic changes

SPINA BIFIDA OCCULTA

Incomplete closure of one or more vertebrae without protrusion of spinal cord or meninges ➡	Skin abnormalities over spinal defect: depression or dimple, tuft of hair, soft fatty deposits, port wine nevi

SPINA BIFIDA CYSTICA

Incomplete closure of one or more vertebrae without protrusion of spinal contents ➡	Saclike structure protruding over spine, trophic skin disturbances, ulcerations
Spinal nerve roots ending at sac ➡	Neurologic dysfunction, possibly including spastic paralysis and bowel and bladder incontinence

TYPES OF SPINA BIFIDA

SPINA BIFIDA OCCULTA

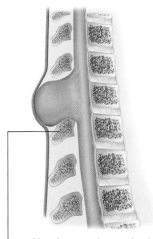

Vertebrae are incompletely fused; no external sac is present.

MENINGOCELE

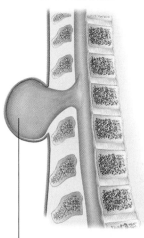

External sac contains meninges and cere-brospinal fluid (CSF).

MYELOMENINGOCELE

External sac contains meninges, CSF, peripheral nerves, and spinal cord tissue.

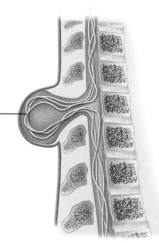

Spinal cord injury

- Fractures, contusions, and compressions of the vertebral column
- Usually results from trauma to the head or neck
- May involve entire spinal cord or affect only one-half of the cord; may occur at any vertebral level

Causes
- Falls
- Gunshot or stab wounds
- Hyperparathyroidism
- Lifting heavy objects
- Motor vehicle accidents
- Neoplastic lesions
- Sports injuries or diving

Pathophysiologic changes

Complete cord transection ➤	Tetraplegia, muscle flaccidity, loss of all reflexes and sensory function below level of injury, bladder and bowel atony, paralytic ileus, unstable blood pressure, dry skin, respiratory impairment
Incomplete cord transection ➤	Motor deficits, variable degree of bladder dysfunction, sensorimotor dysfunction

EFFECTS OF SPINAL CORD INJURY

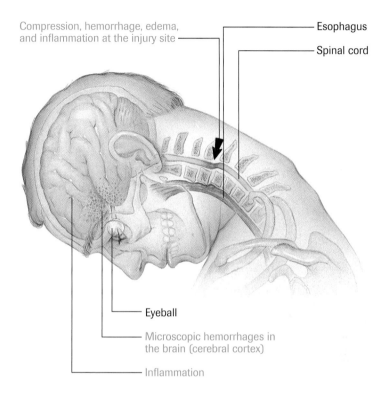

Compression, hemorrhage, edema, and inflammation at the injury site

Esophagus

Spinal cord

Eyeball

Microscopic hemorrhages in the brain (cerebral cortex)

Inflammation

Stroke

- Sudden impairment of cerebral circulation in one or more blood vessels
- Symptoms varied according to affected artery, severity of damage, and extent of collateral circulation
- Stroke in one hemisphere: effects on opposite side of body
- Stroke that damages cranial nerves: effects on same side of body

Causes

- Emboli or thrombosis (ischemic stroke)
- Spontaneous bleeding in brain (hemorrhagic stroke)

Pathophysiologic changes

Thrombosis or hemorrhage of middle cerebral artery ➤	Aphasia or dysphasia, visual field deficits, hemiparesis of affected side (more severe in face and arms)
Thrombosis or hemorrhage of carotid artery ➤	Weakness, paralysis, numbness; sensory changes; altered level of consciousness; bruits over carotid artery; headaches
Thrombosis or hemorrhage of vertebrobasilar artery ➤	Weakness, paralysis; numbness around lips and mouth; visual field deficits, diplopia, nystagmus; poor coordination, dizziness; dysphagia, slurred speech; amnesia; ataxia
Thrombosis or hemorrhage of anterior cerebral artery ➤	Confusion; weakness, numbness; urinary incontinence; impaired motor and sensory functions; personality changes
Thrombosis or hemorrhage of posterior cerebral artery ➤	Visual field deficits; sensory impairment; dyslexia; cortical blindness; coma

ISCHEMIC STROKE

COMMON SITES OF CARDIAC THROMBOSIS

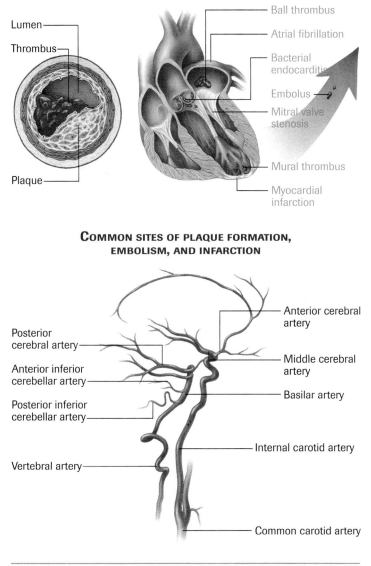

Lumen

Thrombus

Plaque

Ball thrombus

Atrial fibrillation

Bacterial endocarditis

Embolus

Mitral valve stenosis

Mural thrombus

Myocardial infarction

COMMON SITES OF PLAQUE FORMATION, EMBOLISM, AND INFARCTION

Posterior cerebral artery

Anterior inferior cerebellar artery

Posterior inferior cerebellar artery

Vertebral artery

Anterior cerebral artery

Middle cerebral artery

Basilar artery

Internal carotid artery

Common carotid artery

West Nile encephalitis

- Vector-borne infectious disease primarily causing encephalitis of the brain
- Caused by West Nile virus, a flavivirus (type of mosquito or tick-borne virus that causes yellow fever and malaria) commonly found in humans, birds, and other vertebrates
- Mortality rate ranging from 3% to 15% (higher among elderly population)

Causes
- Bite by infected mosquito (primarily *Culex* species)
- Possibly through bite by infected tick

Pathophysiologic changes

Transmission of virus into bloodstream following mosquito bite ➤	Mild infection: flulike symptoms (fever, headache, body aches), swollen lymph glands, skin rash
Inflammation of brain and spinal cord (occurs as virus travels to nervous system) ➤	Severe infection leading to encephalitis: headache, high fever, neck stiffness, stupor, disorientation, coma, tremors, occasional seizures, paralysis

CEREBRAL EDEMA IN WEST NILE VIRUS

NORMAL BRAIN

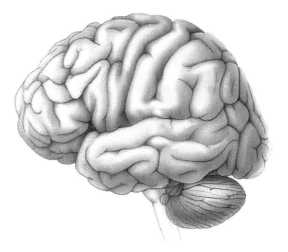

EDEMATOUS BRAIN

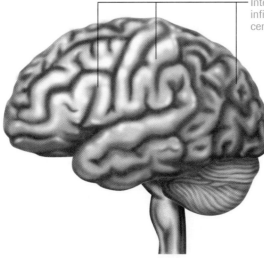

Intense lymphocytic infiltration causing cerebral edema

4

Gastrointestinal system

Appendicitis

- Inflammation and obstruction of the vermiform appendix
- Most common major surgical disease
- Incidence and death rate decreased by antibiotics
- Untreated, invariably fatal

Causes
- Barium ingestion
- Fecal mass
- Foreign body
- Mucosal ulceration
- Neoplasm
- Stricture
- Viral infection

Pathophysiologic changes

Bowel obstruction and distention ➧	Abdominal pain, anorexia
Inflammation and pressure ➧	Pain, nausea, vomiting, low-grade fever, tenderness

APPENDIX OBSTRUCTION AND INFLAMMATION

SMALL AND LARGE INTESTINES

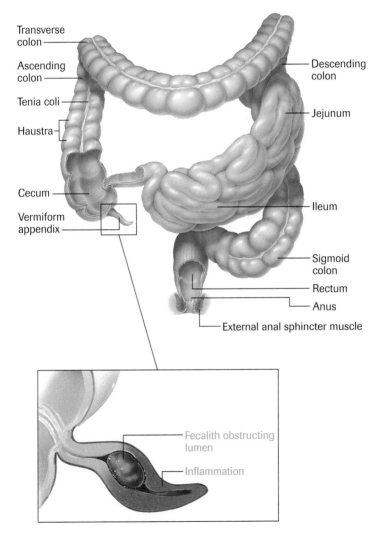

Transverse colon

Ascending colon

Tenia coli

Haustra

Cecum

Vermiform appendix

Descending colon

Jejunum

Ileum

Sigmoid colon

Rectum

Anus

External anal sphincter muscle

Fecalith obstructing lumen

Inflammation

Cholecystitis

- Acute or chronic inflammation causing painful distention of the gallbladder
- Usually associated with a gallstone impacted in the cystic duct
- Good prognosis with treatment

Causes
- Abnormal metabolism of bile salts and cholesterol
- Gallstones
- Poor or absent blood flow to the gallbladder

Pathophysiologic changes

Infection and inflammation of nerve fibers ➡	Acute abdominal pain in the right upper quadrant that may radiate to the back, between the shoulders, or to the front of the chest; nausea, vomiting and chills
Passage of gallstones along the bile duct ➡	Colic, jaundice if obstruction

SITES OF GALLSTONES

LIVER AND GALLBLADDER

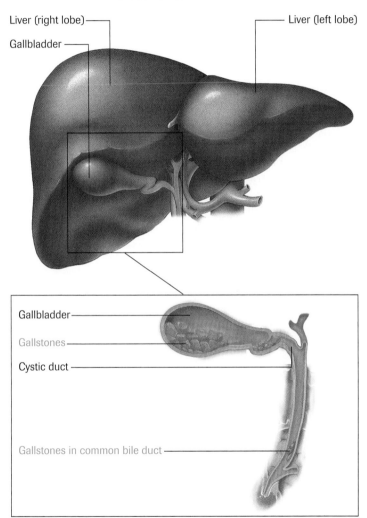

Liver (right lobe)
Liver (left lobe)
Gallbladder

Gallbladder
Gallstones
Cystic duct

Gallstones in common bile duct

Cirrhosis

- Chronic disease characterized by diffuse destruction and fibrotic degeneration of hepatic cells
- Damages liver tissue and normal vasculature
- Especially prevalent among malnourished people older than age 50 with chronic alcoholism

Causes

- Alcoholism
- Alpha$_1$-antitrypsin deficiency
- Biliary obstruction
- Budd-Chiari syndrome
- Hemochromatosis
- Hepatitis
- Wilson's disease

Pathophysiologic changes

Fibrotic changes ▶	Hepatomegaly
Gastric stasis ▶	Anorexia
Inflammatory response and systemic effects of liver inflammation ▶	Nausea and vomiting, dull abdominal ache
Fluid retention ▶	Edema and ascites
Impaired liver function ▶	Jaundice
Portal hypertension ▶	Esophageal varices

CIRRHOTIC CHANGES

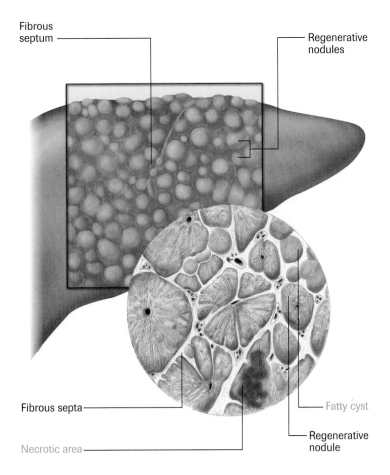

Fibrous septum

Regenerative nodules

Fibrous septa

Necrotic area

Fatty cyst

Regenerative nodule

Colonic polyps

- Small tumorlike growths projecting from the mucosal surface of the colon
- Types: common polypoid adenomas, villous adenomas, hereditary polyposis, focal polypoid hyperplasia, juvenile polyps
- Most benign; however, villous and hereditary polyps tending to become malignant
- Juvenile polyps: characterized by rectal bleeding
- Familial polyps: strong association with rectosigmoid adenocarcinoma

Causes

- Unknown
- Predisposing factors: age, diet, heredity, infection, sedentary lifestyle

Pathophysiologic changes

Unrestrained cell growth in the upper epithelium of the colon ➤	Masses of tissue protruding into the GI tract
Bleeding polyps ➤	High polyps leave a streak of blood on the stool; low rectal polyps bleed freely
Cell growth into the GI tract ➤	Painful defecation, diarrhea

POLYPS WITHIN THE COLON

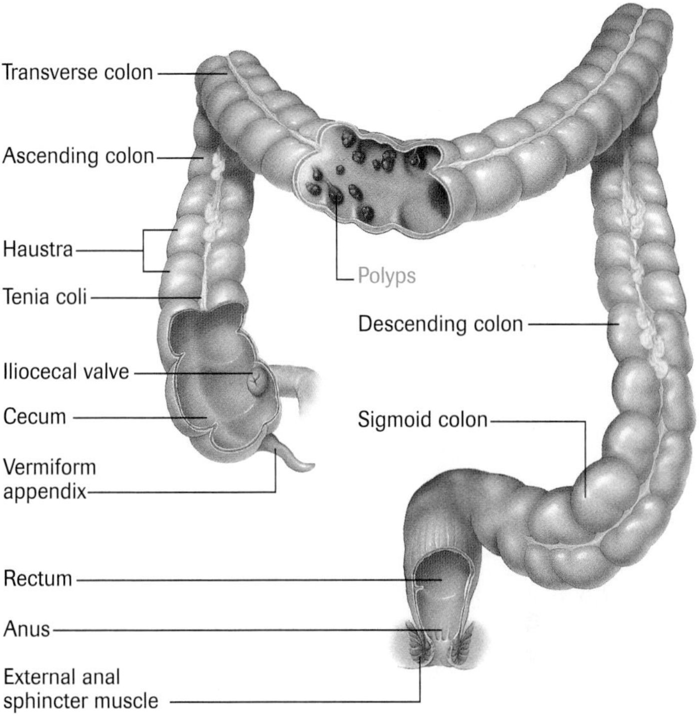

Transverse colon

Ascending colon

Haustra

Tenia coli

Polyps

Descending colon

Iliocecal valve

Cecum

Sigmoid colon

Vermiform appendix

Rectum

Anus

External anal sphincter muscle

Colorectal cancer

- Slow-growing cancer that usually starts in the inner layer of intestinal tract
- Commonly begins as polyp
- Signs and symptoms dependend on location of tumor
- Potentially curable if diagnosed early

Causes
- Unknown

Pathophysiologic changes

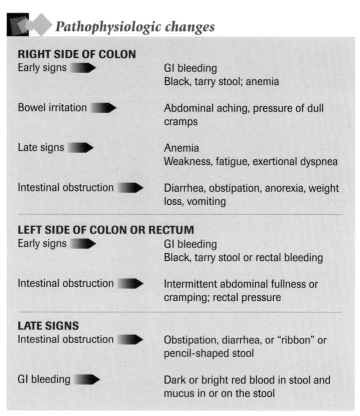

RIGHT SIDE OF COLON

Early signs ➤	GI bleeding Black, tarry stool; anemia
Bowel irritation ➤	Abdominal aching, pressure of dull cramps
Late signs ➤	Anemia Weakness, fatigue, exertional dyspnea
Intestinal obstruction ➤	Diarrhea, obstipation, anorexia, weight loss, vomiting

LEFT SIDE OF COLON OR RECTUM

Early signs ➤	GI bleeding Black, tarry stool or rectal bleeding
Intestinal obstruction ➤	Intermittent abdominal fullness or cramping; rectal pressure

LATE SIGNS

Intestinal obstruction ➤	Obstipation, diarrhea, or "ribbon" or pencil-shaped stool
GI bleeding ➤	Dark or bright red blood in stool and mucus in or on the stool

TYPES OF COLORECTAL CANCER

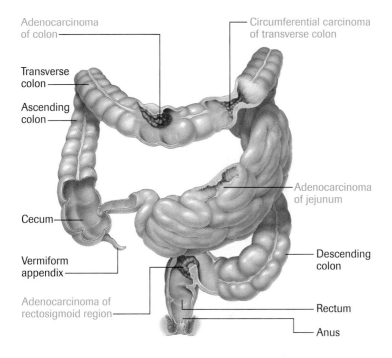

Adenocarcinoma of colon

Circumferential carcinoma of transverse colon

Transverse colon

Ascending colon

Adenocarcinoma of jejunum

Cecum

Descending colon

Vermiform appendix

Adenocarcinoma of rectosigmoid region

Rectum

Anus

Crohn's disease

- Slowly spreading, progressive inflammatory bowel disease
- Involves any part of the GI tract, usually proximal portion of colon; also may affect terminal ileum
- Expands through all layers of intestinal wall
- Causes thickening and narrowing of bowel lumen, leading to malabsorption and intestinal obstruction

Causes
- Unknown
- Possibly, immune reaction to virus or bacterium that causes ongoing intestinal inflammation

Pathophysiologic changes

Loss of absorptive surface of functional mucosa ➡	Protein-calorie malnutrition, dehydration, and nutritional deficiencies; weight loss; diarrhea; steatorrhea
Edema of mucosa and bowel spasm ➡	Obstruction of small or large intestine
Bowel spasm ➡	Steady, colicky pain in right lower quadrant; cramping; tenderness
Thickened or matted loops of inflamed bowel ➡	Palpable mass in right lower quadrant
Inflammation ➡	Bloody stools

BOWEL CHANGES IN CROHN'S DISEASE

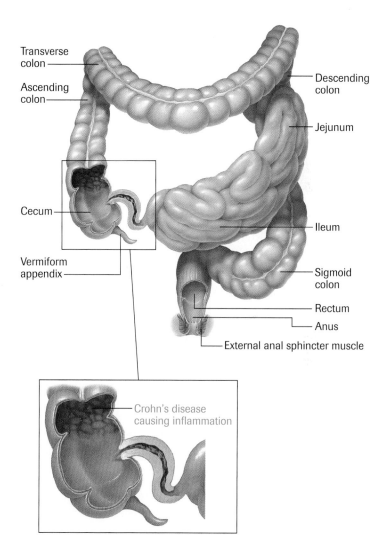

Transverse colon

Ascending colon

Cecum

Vermiform appendix

Descending colon

Jejunum

Ileum

Sigmoid colon

Rectum

Anus

External anal sphincter muscle

Crohn's disease causing inflammation

Diverticular disease

- Characterized by bulging pouches in GI wall that push mucosal lining through surrounding muscle
- Classified as diverticulosis (diverticula are present but don't cause symptoms) or diverticulitis (diverticula that are inflamed; may cause potentially fatal obstruction, infection, or hemorrhage)

Causes
- Defects in colon wall strength
- Diminished colonic motility and increased intraluminal pressure
- Low-fiber diet

Pathophysiologic changes

MILD DIVERTICULITIS

Inflammation of diverticula ➤ Moderate left lower abdominal pain

Trapping of bacteria-rich stool in diverticula ➤ Low-grade fever, leukocytosis

SEVERE DIVERTICULITIS

Rupture of diverticula and subsequent inflammation and infection ➤ Abdominal rigidity, left lower quadrant pain

Sepsis ➤ High fever, chills, hypotension

Rupture of diverticula near vessel ➤ Microscopic or massive hemorrhage

CHRONIC DIVERTICULITIS

Intestinal obstruction ➤ Constipation; ribbon-like stools; intermittent diarrhea; abdominal distention, rigidity, and pain; diminishing or absent bowel sounds; nausea and vomiting

DIVERTICULOSIS OF THE COLON

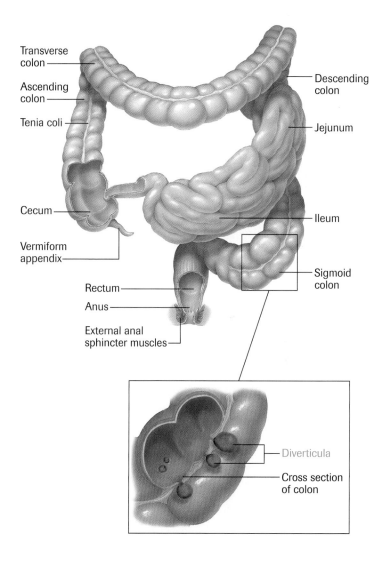

Transverse colon

Ascending colon

Tenia coli

Cecum

Vermiform appendix

Descending colon

Jejunum

Ileum

Sigmoid colon

Rectum

Anus

External anal sphincter muscles

Diverticula

Cross section of colon

Esophageal cancer

- Usually fatal type of cancer
- Two types of malignant tumors: squamous cell carcinoma and adenocarcinoma
- Common sites of distant metastasis: liver, lungs
- Incidence greater in Japan, China, the Middle East, and parts of South Africa

Causes

- Unknown
- Predisposing factors: excessive alcohol use and heavy smoking, diets high in nitrosamines, history of head and neck tumors, nutritional deficiencies, stasis induced inflammation

Pathophysiologic changes

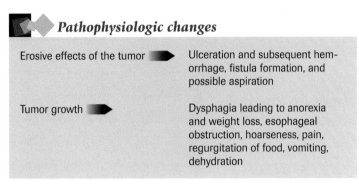

Erosive effects of the tumor ➤	Ulceration and subsequent hemorrhage, fistula formation, and possible aspiration
Tumor growth ➤	Dysphagia leading to anorexia and weight loss, esophageal obstruction, hoarseness, pain, regurgitation of food, vomiting, dehydration

COMMON ESOPHAGEAL CANCERS

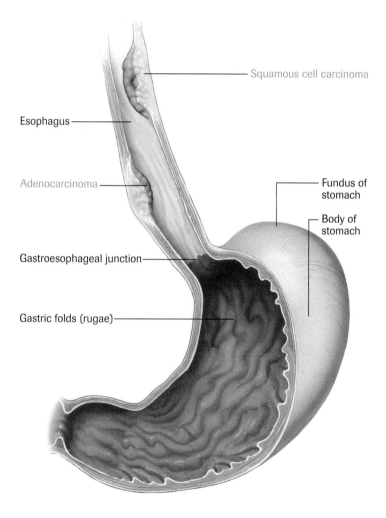

Squamous cell carcinoma

Esophagus

Adenocarcinoma

Gastroesophageal junction

Gastric folds (rugae)

Fundus of stomach

Body of stomach

Gastric cancer

- Classified as polyploid, ulcerating, ulcerating and infiltrating, or diffuse
- Infiltrates rapidly to regional lymph nodes, omentum, liver, and lungs
- Common throughout the world, but mortality highest in Japan, Iceland, Chile, and Austria

Causes
- Unknown, but commonly associated with atrophic gastritis
- Predisposing factors: asbestos exposure, eating pickled or smoked foods, family history, *Helicobacter pylori* infection, high alcohol intake, smoking, type A blood

Pathophysiologic changes

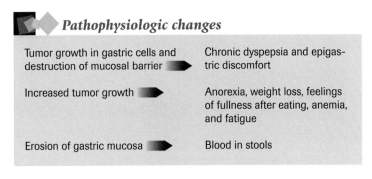

Tumor growth in gastric cells and destruction of mucosal barrier ➤	Chronic dyspepsia and epigastric discomfort
Increased tumor growth ➤	Anorexia, weight loss, feelings of fullness after eating, anemia, and fatigue
Erosion of gastric mucosa ➤	Blood in stools

ADENOCARCINOMA OF THE STOMACH

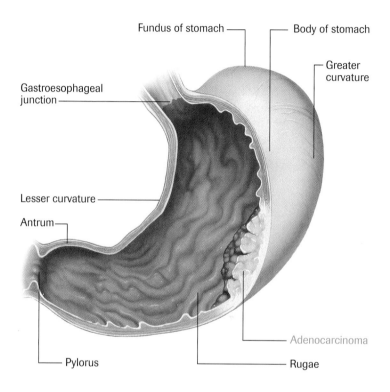

Fundus of stomach

Body of stomach

Greater curvature

Gastroesophageal junction

Lesser curvature

Antrum

Adenocarcinoma

Pylorus

Rugae

Gastritis

- Acute or chronic inflammation of the gastric mucosa that's benign and self-limiting
- Usually a response to local irritants
- Chronic gastritis common among elderly people and individuals with pernicious anemia

Causes
ACUTE GASTRITIS
- Bacterial endotoxins
- Ingestion of irritants, certain medications, and poisons
- Physiologic stress

CHRONIC GASTRITIS
- Diabetes mellitus
- *Helicobacter pylori* infection
- Peptic ulcer disease
- Pernicious anemia
- Renal disease

Pathophysiologic changes

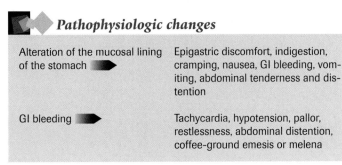

Alteration of the mucosal lining of the stomach ➤	Epigastric discomfort, indigestion, cramping, nausea, GI bleeding, vomiting, abdominal tenderness and distention
GI bleeding ➤	Tachycardia, hypotension, pallor, restlessness, abdominal distention, coffee-ground emesis or melena

ACUTE GASTRITIS

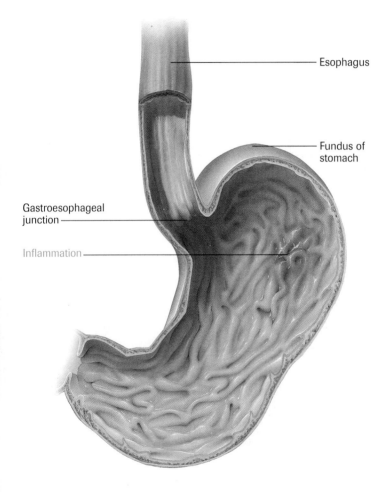

Esophagus

Fundus of stomach

Gastroesophageal junction

Inflammation

Gastroesophageal reflux

- Backflow of gastric or duodenal contents (or both) into the esophagus and past the lower esophageal sphincter (LES), without associated belching or vomiting
- Causes acute epigastric pain, usually after meals

Causes
- Alcohol, cigarettes, or food, causing LES pressure
- Hiatal hernia
- Increased abdominal pressure (obesity, pregnancy)
- Medications
- Nasogastric intubation for more than 4 days
- Weakened esophageal sphincter

Pathophysiologic changes

Increased abdominal pressure and esophageal irritation ➡	Burning pain in epigastric area (usually following meals or when lying down)
Stomach contents flow into the esophagus ➡	Feeling of fluid accumulation in the throat, sour or bitter taste in the mouth, dyspepsia, nausea and vomiting

UNDERSTANDING
GASTROESOPHAGEAL REFLUX

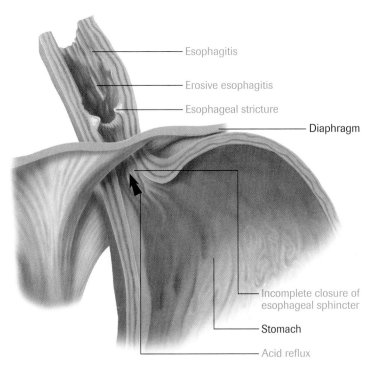

Esophagitis

Erosive esophagitis

Esophageal stricture

Diaphragm

Incomplete closure of esophageal sphincter

Stomach

Acid reflux

Hemorrhoids

- Painful, swollen vein in the lower portion of the rectum or anus
- Common; especially occurs during pregnancy and after childbirth
- Results from increased pressure in the veins of the anus, causing them to bulge and expand

Causes

- Constipation, low-fiber diet, straining at defecation
- Obesity
- Pregnancy
- Prolonged sitting

Pathophysiologic changes

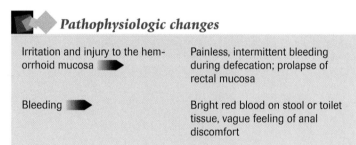

Irritation and injury to the hemorrhoid mucosa ➤	Painless, intermittent bleeding during defecation; prolapse of rectal mucosa
Bleeding ➤	Bright red blood on stool or toilet tissue, vague feeling of anal discomfort

INTERNAL AND EXTERNAL HEMORRHOIDS

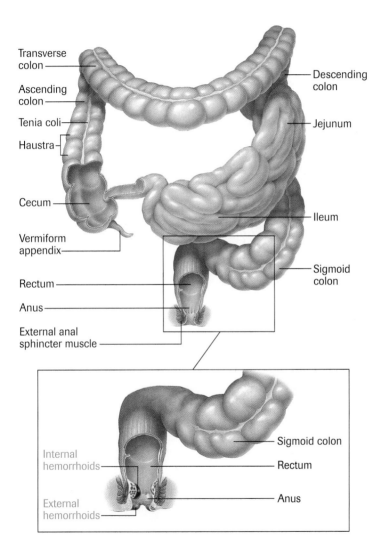

Transverse colon

Descending colon

Ascending colon

Tenia coli

Jejunum

Haustra

Cecum

Ileum

Vermiform appendix

Rectum

Sigmoid colon

Anus

External anal sphincter muscle

Internal hemorrhoids

Sigmoid colon

Rectum

External hemorrhoids

Anus

Hepatitis, viral

- Common liver infection that causes hepatic cell destruction, necrosis, and autolysis
- Major types differentiated by causative virus and transmission
- Type A: highly contagious; usually resulting from ingestion of contaminated food or water
- Type B: spread through contact with contaminated blood, secretions, and stool
- Type C: blood-borne disease associated with shared needles, blood transfusions
- Type D: linked to chronic hepatitis B infection; can be severe and lead to fulminant hepatitis
- Type E: associated with recent travel to endemic area

Cause
- Infection with causative virus

Pathophysiologic changes

PRODROMAL STAGE

Systemic effects of inflammation ▶	Fatigue, malaise, arthralgia, myalgia, fever
Anorexia ▶	Mild weight loss
Liver inflammation ▶	Nausea and vomiting, changes in senses of taste and smell, right upper quadrant tenderness
Urobilinogen ▶	Dark colored urine
Decreased bile in GI tract ▶	Clay-colored stools

CLINICAL STAGE
Characterized by worsening of all symptoms of prodromal stage

Increased bilirubin in blood ▶	Itching, jaundice
Continued liver inflammation ▶	Abdominal pain or tenderness

RECOVERY STAGE
Characterized by subsiding of symptoms and returning of appetite

UNDERSTANDING LIVER BIOPSY RESULTS

NORMAL BIOPSY

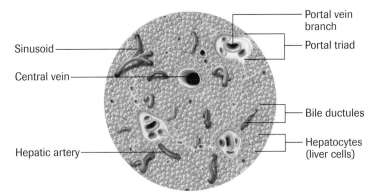

Sinusoid

Central vein

Hepatic artery

Portal vein branch

Portal triad

Bile ductules

Hepatocytes (liver cells)

MILD HEPATITIS

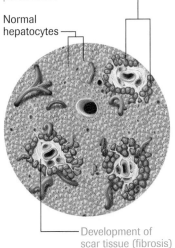

Mild swelling and inflammation of damaged liver cells around portal areas

Normal hepatocytes

Development of scar tissue (fibrosis)

MODERATE HEPATITIS

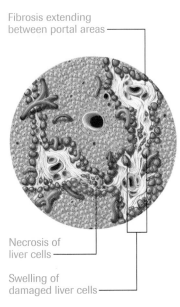

Fibrosis extending between portal areas

Necrosis of liver cells

Swelling of damaged liver cells

Hiatal hernia

- Defect in the diaphragm that permits a portion of the stomach to pass through the diaphragmatic opening into the chest
- Most common problem of the diaphragm affecting the alimentary canal

Causes
- Congenital diaphragm malformations
- Esophageal carcinoma
- Kyphoscoliosis
- Trauma

Pathophysiologic changes

Increased intra-abdominal pressure ➤	Heartburn 1 to 4 hours after eating, regurgitation or vomiting, retrosternal or substernal chest pain, dysphagia, feeling of fullness after eating

STOMACH HERNIATION

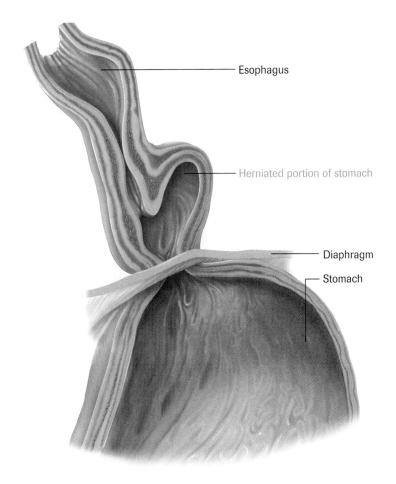

Esophagus

Herniated portion of stomach

Diaphragm

Stomach

Hirschsprung's disease

- Congenital disorder of large intestine
- Characterized by absence or marked reduction of parasympathetic ganglion cells in the colorectal wall
- Usually coexisting with other congenital anomalies

Causes
- Familial congenital defect

Pathophysiologic changes

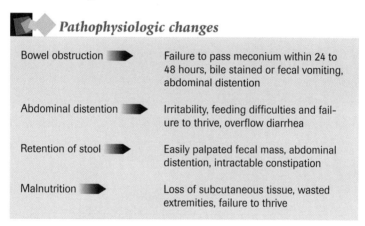

Bowel obstruction ➤	Failure to pass meconium within 24 to 48 hours, bile stained or fecal vomiting, abdominal distention
Abdominal distention ➤	Irritability, feeding difficulties and failure to thrive, overflow diarrhea
Retention of stool ➤	Easily palpated fecal mass, abdominal distention, intractable constipation
Malnutrition ➤	Loss of subcutaneous tissue, wasted extremities, failure to thrive

BOWEL DILATION IN
HIRSCHSPRUNG'S DISEASE

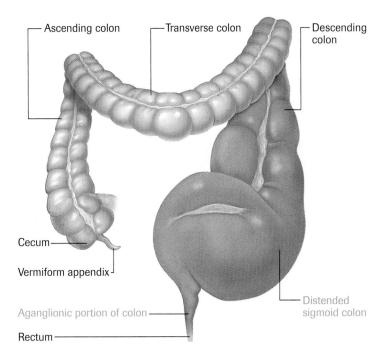

Ascending colon

Transverse colon

Descending colon

Cecum

Vermiform appendix

Aganglionic portion of colon

Rectum

Distended sigmoid colon

Inguinal hernia

- Occurs in the large or small intestine, omentum, or bladder and protruding into the inguinal canal
- In infants, commonly coexists with an undescended testicle or hydrocele

Causes
- Increased intra-abdominal pressure
- Weak abdominal muscles
- Weak fascial floor of inguinal canal
- Weak fascial margin of internal inguinal ring

Pathophysiologic changes

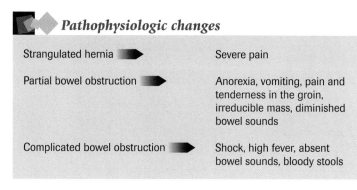

Strangulated hernia ➤	Severe pain
Partial bowel obstruction ➤	Anorexia, vomiting, pain and tenderness in the groin, irreducible mass, diminished bowel sounds
Complicated bowel obstruction ➤	Shock, high fever, absent bowel sounds, bloody stools

INDIRECT INGUINAL HERNIA

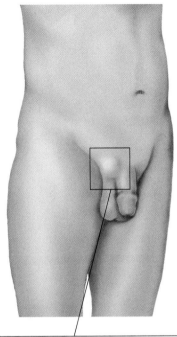

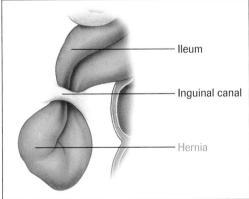

Ileum

Inguinal canal

Hernia

Irritable bowel syndrome

- Benign condition that has no anatomical abnormality or inflammatory component
- Marked by chronic symptoms of abdominal pain, alternating constipation and diarrhea, excess flatus, sense of incomplete evacuation, and abdominal distention
- Common, stress-related disorder

Causes
- Abuse of laxatives
- Hormonal changes (menstruation)
- Ingestion of irritants (coffee, raw fruit or vegetables)
- Lactose intolerance
- Psychological stress (most common)

Pathophysiologic changes

Muscle contraction ➤	Cramping, lower abdominal pain relieved by defecation or passage of flatus
Irritation of nerve fibers by causative stimulus ➤	Pain that intensifies 1 to 2 hours after a meal
Altered colonic movement ➤	Constipation alternating with diarrhea, mucus passed through rectum from altered secretion in the intestinal lumen, abdominal distention and bloating

EFFECTS OF IRRITABLE BOWEL SYNDROME

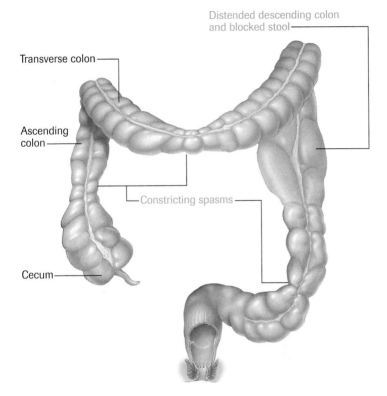

Distended descending colon and blocked stool

Transverse colon

Ascending colon

Cecum

Constricting spasms

Liver cancer

- Rare form of primary cancer in the United States
- Rapidly fatal, usually within 6 months from GI hemorrhage, progressive cachexia, liver failure, or metastasis
- Common for patients with hepatomas to have cirrhosis

Causes
- Immediate cause unknown
- Possibly congenital in children

Pathophysiologic changes

Mutation in cells of liver tissue ➤	Mass or enlargement in right upper quadrant; tender, nodular liver on palpation; severe epigastric or right upper quadrant pain; bruit, hum or rubbing sound with large tumor
Blockage of bile duct ➤	Jaundice, ascites, anorexia
Increased tumor growth needs ➤	Weight loss, anorexia, nausea, vomiting, malaise, weakness

COMMON SITES OF LIVER CANCER

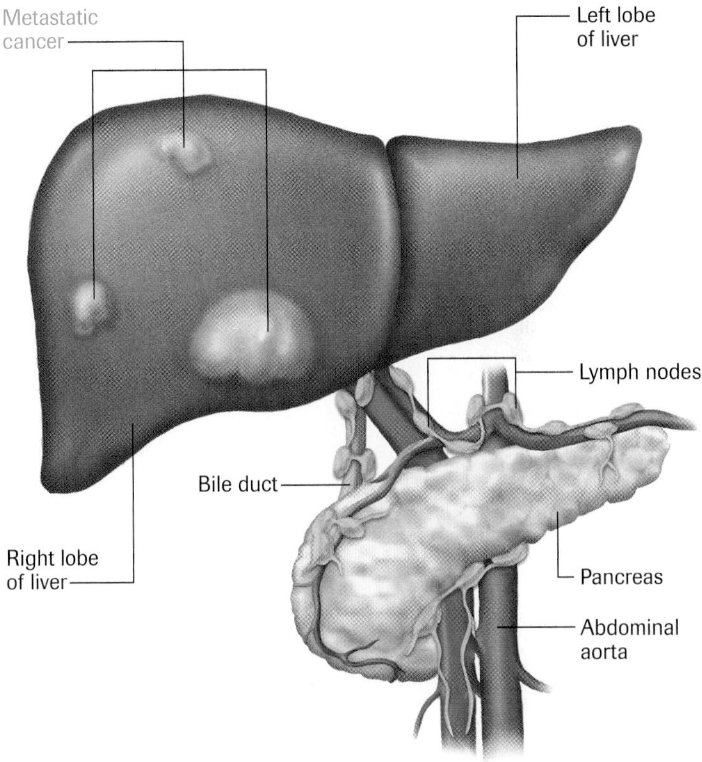

Metastatic cancer

Left lobe of liver

Lymph nodes

Bile duct

Right lobe of liver

Pancreas

Abdominal aorta

Pancreatic cancer

- Occurs primarily in the head of the organ
- Progresses to death within 1 year of diagnosis
- Fourth leading cause of cancer deaths in the United States

Causes
- Inhalation or absorption of carcinogens, which are excreted by the pancreas (cigarette smoke, food additives, industrial chemicals)

Pathophysiologic changes

Obstruction of bile flow ➡	Jaundice, clay-colored stools, dark urine
Duodenal obstruction ➡	Nausea and vomiting
Tumor cytokines acting as platelet aggregating factors ➡	Recurrent thrombophlebitis
Increased tumor growth needs ➡	Weight loss, anorexia, malaise
Tumor growth and pressure ➡	Abdominal or back pain

PANCREATIC ADENOCARCINOMA

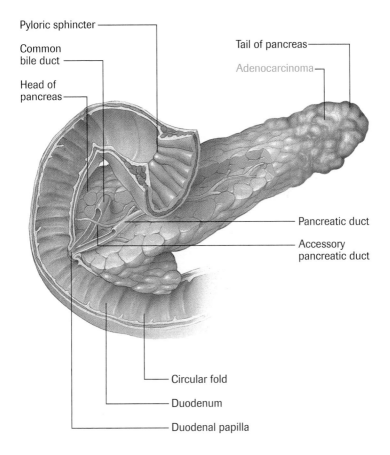

Pyloric sphincter

Common
bile duct

Head of
pancreas

Tail of pancreas

Adenocarcinoma

Pancreatic duct

Accessory
pancreatic duct

Circular fold

Duodenum

Duodenal papilla

Pancreatitis

- Inflammation of the pancreas; occurring in acute and chronic forms
- May be caused by edema, necrosis, or hemorrhage
- Good prognosis when associated with biliary tract disease; poor when associated with alcoholism
- Mortality as high as 60% with necrosis and hemorrhage

Causes

- Acute pancreatitis: abnormal organ structure, alcohol abuse, blunt or surgical trauma, cholelithiasis, drugs, endocrine or metabolic disorders, kidney failure or transplantation, pancreatic cysts or tumors, penetrating peptic ulcers
- Chronic pancreatitis: alcohol abuse, heredity, malnutrition

Pathophysiologic changes

Inflammation ➤	Midepigastric abdominal pain; low-grade fever
Hypermotility or paralytic ileus secondary to pancreatitis or peritonitis ➤	Persistent vomiting and abdominal distention (in a severe attack)
Heart failure ➤	Crackles at lung bases (in severe attack)
Circulating pancreatic enzymes ➤	Left pleural effusion (in severe attack)
Dehydration and possible hypovolemia ➤	Tachycardia
Malabsorption ➤	Extreme malaise (in chronic pancreatitis)

NECROTIZING PANCREATITIS

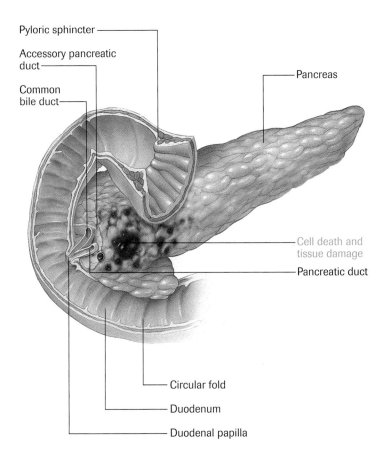

Pyloric sphincter

Accessory pancreatic duct

Common bile duct

Pancreas

Cell death and tissue damage

Pancreatic duct

Circular fold

Duodenum

Duodenal papilla

Peritonitis

- Acute or chronic inflammation of the peritoneum
- Inflammation possibly extending throughout the peritoneum or localized as an abscess
- With antibiotic treatment, mortality rate 10% (usually related to bowel obstruction)

Causes
- Abdominal neoplasm
- Appendicitis, diverticulitis
- Chronic liver disease
- Penetrating trauma
- Peptic ulcer, ulcerative colitis
- Perforation of gastric ulcer
- Released pancreatic enzymes
- Renal failure
- Rupture of the bladder or fallopian tube
- Volvulus, strangulated obstruction

Pathophysiologic changes

Inflammation and infectious processes ➤	Severe abdominal pain, rigid abdomen, fever, cloudy peritoneal dialysis fluid, nausea, vomiting
Translocation of extracellular fluid into the peritoneal cavity ➤	Tachycardia, hypotension, shock, dehydration, pallor, diaphoresis, cold skin
Irritation of the phrenic nerve ➤	Hiccups

GENERALIZED PERITONITIS

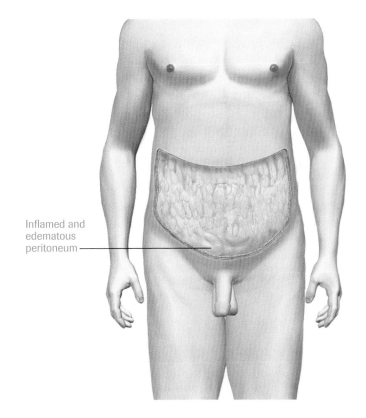

Inflamed and
edematous
peritoneum

Portal hypertension

- Induced by an increased resistance to blood flow through the liver
- Limited blood flow causing splanchnic arterial flow to increase
- Results in overloading of the portal system from elevated pressure in the portal veins
- Decreases liver's ability to remove waste products from the blood and toxins accumulating within the body

Causes
- Budd-Chiari syndrome (mechanical obstruction and occlusion of the hepatic veins)
- Cirrhosis

Pathophysiologic changes

Portosystemic shunting of blood	Esophageal varices, hemorrhoids, or prominent abdominal veins
Increased pressure in the peritoneal capillaries	Ascites, splenomegaly
Splenomegaly	Anemia, leukopenia, thrombocytopenia
Ascites	Fluid retention, edema of the legs, increased abdominal girth, decreased plasma proteins
Blood clotting deficiencies	Acute GI bleeding, thrombocytopenia, bleeding esophageal varices, anemia, easy bruising, bleeding gums, nosebleeds
Shunting of ammonia and toxins into the general circulation	Mental confusion, lethargy, slurred speech, hallucinations, paranoia, coma

PORTAL HYPERTENSION AND VARICES

Increased pressure stimulates the development of collateral channels (varices), which attempt to bypass the portal vein flow into the liver.

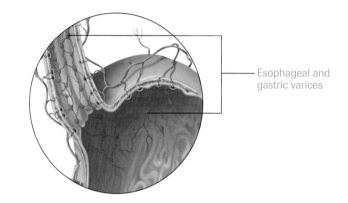

Esophageal and gastric varices

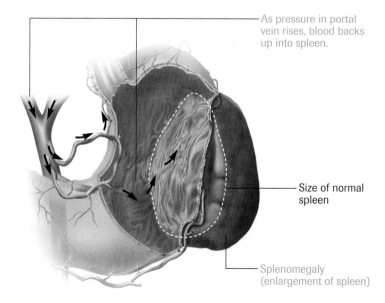

As pressure in portal vein rises, blood backs up into spleen.

Size of normal spleen

Splenomegaly (enlargement of spleen)

Pyloric stenosis

- Narrowing of the pylorus, the outlet from the stomach to the small intestine
- Occurs primarily in infants; rare in patients older than age 6 months
- More common in girls than boys

Causes
- Unknown, possibly related to genetic factors

Pathophysiologic changes

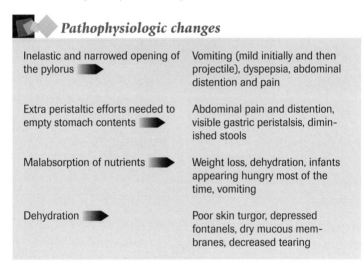

Inelastic and narrowed opening of the pylorus ➡	Vomiting (mild initially and then projectile), dyspepsia, abdominal distention and pain
Extra peristaltic efforts needed to empty stomach contents ➡	Abdominal pain and distention, visible gastric peristalsis, diminished stools
Malabsorption of nutrients ➡	Weight loss, dehydration, infants appearing hungry most of the time, vomiting
Dehydration ➡	Poor skin turgor, depressed fontanels, dry mucous membranes, decreased tearing

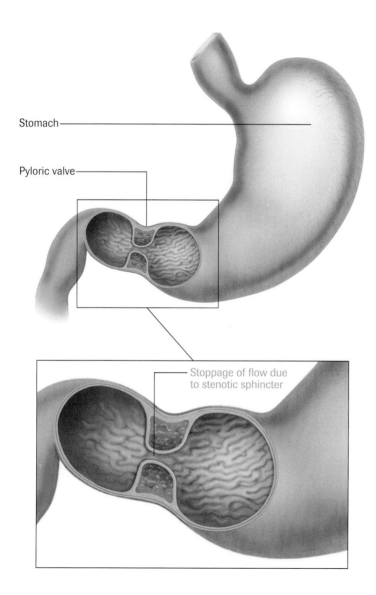

Stomach

Pyloric valve

Stoppage of flow due to stenotic sphincter

Ulcerative colitis

- Continuous inflammatory disease affecting the mucosa of the colon and rectum
- Begins in the rectum and sigmoid colon and extending upward into the entire colon
- Commonly produces edema and ulcerations
- Cycles of exacerbation and remission

Causes

- Unknown
- May be related to abnormal immune response to food or bacteria such as *Escherichia coli*

Pathophysiologic changes

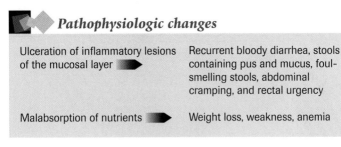

Ulceration of inflammatory lesions of the mucosal layer ➤	Recurrent bloody diarrhea, stools containing pus and mucus, foul-smelling stools, abdominal cramping, and rectal urgency
Malabsorption of nutrients ➤	Weight loss, weakness, anemia

MUCOSAL CHANGES IN ULCERATIVE COLITIS

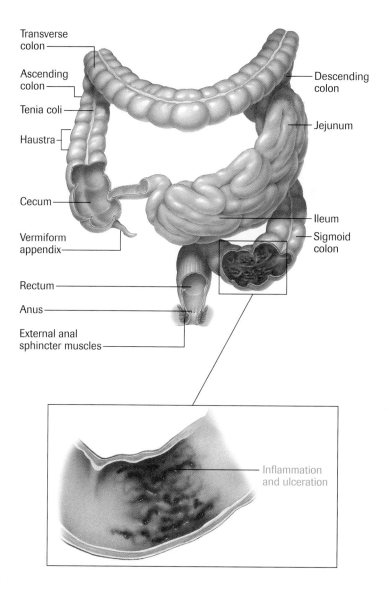

Transverse colon

Ascending colon

Tenia coli

Haustra

Cecum

Vermiform appendix

Rectum

Anus

External anal sphincter muscles

Descending colon

Jejunum

Ileum

Sigmoid colon

Inflammation and ulceration

Ulcers

- Circumscribed lesions in the mucosal membrane extending below the epithelium
- May develop in the lower esophagus, stomach, pylorus, duodenum, and jejunum
- Acute or chronic
- Acute ulcers multiple and superficial
- Chronic ulcers identified by scar tissue at their base

Causes

- *Helicobacter pylori* infection
- Inadequate protection of mucous membrane
- Nonsteroidal anti-inflammatory drugs
- Pathologic hypersecretory disorders

Pathophysiologic changes

GASTRIC ULCER

Decrease in gastric mucosal barrier ➤	Pain that worsens with eating, nausea and anorexia, epigastric tenderness, hyperactive bowel sounds
Pain with eating ➤	Loss of appetite, weight loss

DUODENAL ULCER

Excessive production of acid in the duodenum ➤	Epigastric pain, pain relieved by food or antacids, epigastric tenderness, hyperactive bowel sounds

COMMON ULCER TYPES AND SITES

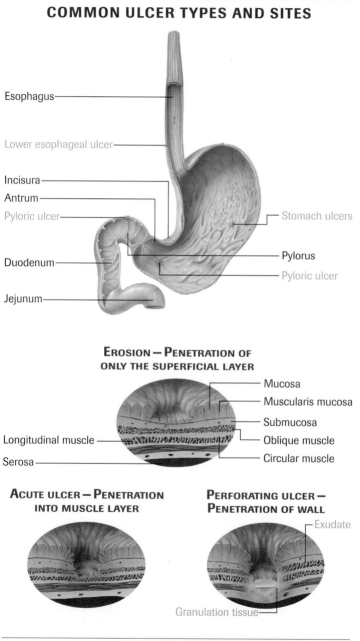

Esophagus

Lower esophageal ulcer

Incisura

Antrum

Pyloric ulcer

Duodenum

Jejunum

Stomach ulcers

Pylorus

Pyloric ulcer

EROSION — PENETRATION OF ONLY THE SUPERFICIAL LAYER

Mucosa

Muscularis mucosa

Submucosa

Longitudinal muscle

Oblique muscle

Serosa

Circular muscle

ACUTE ULCER — PENETRATION INTO MUSCLE LAYER

PERFORATING ULCER — PENETRATION OF WALL

Exudate

Granulation tissue

5

Musculoskeletal system

Bone tumors

- Primary bone tumors rare; most are secondary and caused by seeding from a primary site
- Osseous bone tumors: arise from bony structures and include osteogenic sarcoma, parosteal osteogenic sarcoma, chondrosarcoma, and giant cell tumor
- Nonosseous bone tumors: arise from hematopoietic, vascular, and neural tissues and include Ewing's sarcoma, fibrosarcoma, and chordoma

Causes

- No immediately apparent cause in most cases
- Carcinogen exposure
- Genetic abnormalities
- Heredity, excessive radiation therapy, trauma

Pathophysiologic changes

Inflammation within and around bone ➤	Pain
Tumor growth ➤	Palpable mass
Weakened bone structure ➤	Fractures

TYPES OF BONE TUMORS

GIANT CELL TUMOR

CHONDROBLASTOMA

OSTEOGENIC SARCOMA

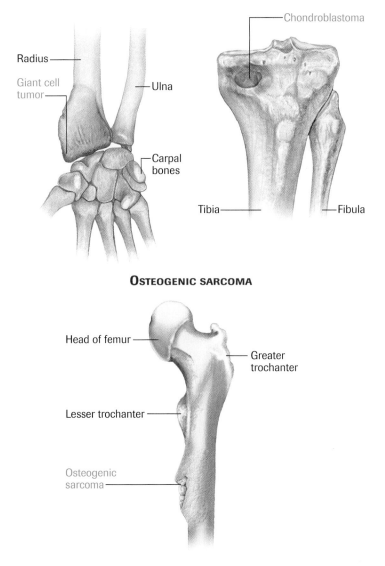

Radius

Giant cell tumor

Ulna

Carpal bones

Chondroblastoma

Tibia

Fibula

Head of femur

Greater trochanter

Lesser trochanter

Osteogenic sarcoma

Bursitis

- Painful inflammation of one or more of the bursae (closed sacs with small amounts of synovial fluid that facilitate the motion of muscles and tendons over bony prominences)
- Usually occurs in the subdeltoid, olecranon, trochanteric, calcaneal, or prepatellar bursae

Causes

- Chronic bursitis (repeated attacks of acute bursitis, infection, or trauma)
- Inflammatory joint disease, such as gout or rheumatoid arthritis
- Recurring trauma that stresses or presses a joint
- Septic bursitis (bacterial invasion of overlying skin; wound infection)

Pathophysiologic changes

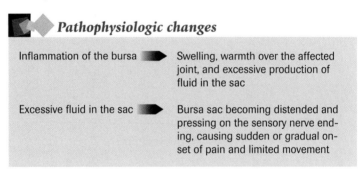

Inflammation of the bursa ➡	Swelling, warmth over the affected joint, and excessive production of fluid in the sac
Excessive fluid in the sac ➡	Bursa sac becoming distended and pressing on the sensory nerve ending, causing sudden or gradual onset of pain and limited movement

BURSITIS OF THE HIP AND KNEE

HIP

Inflamed trochanteric bursae

Head of femur

Neck of femur

Femur

Greater trochanter

KNEE

Quadricep tendon

Inflammation of prepatellar bursa

Patella

Infrapatellar fat pad

Patellar ligament

Femur

Inflammation of deep infrapatellar bursa

Carpal tunnel syndrome

- Compression of median nerve as it passes through canal (tunnel) formed by carpal bones and transverse carpal ligaments
- Most common nerve entrapment syndrome

Causes
- Congenital predisposition
- Development of cyst or tumor within canal
- Fluid retention during menopause or pregnancy
- Hypothyroidism
- Injury or trauma to the wrist
- Mechanical problems in wrist joint
- Obesity
- Overactive pituitary gland
- Rheumatoid arthritis
- Work-related stress

Pathophysiologic changes

Nerve compression ➤	Weakness, pain, burning, numbness, or tingling of thumb, forefinger, middle finger, and half of fourth finger in one or both hands; inability to clench hand into fist
Vasodilation and venous stasis ➤	Worsening of symptoms at night and in the morning

NERVE COMPRESSION IN CARPAL TUNNEL SYNDROME

Cross section of normal wrist

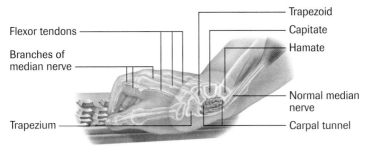

Flexor tendons

Branches of median nerve

Trapezium

Trapezoid

Capitate

Hamate

Normal median nerve

Carpal tunnel

Cross section of wrist with carpal tunnel syndrome

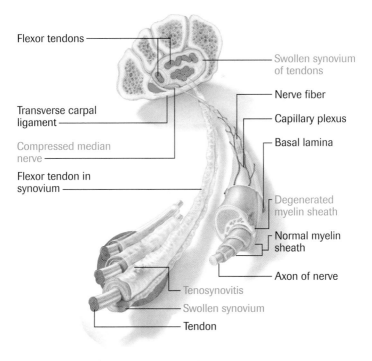

Flexor tendons

Transverse carpal ligament

Compressed median nerve

Flexor tendon in synovium

Swollen synovium of tendons

Nerve fiber

Capillary plexus

Basal lamina

Degenerated myelin sheath

Normal myelin sheath

Axon of nerve

Tenosynovitis

Swollen synovium

Tendon

Developmental dysplasia
of the hip

- Abnormal development or dislocation of the hip joint present from birth
- Most common disorder affecting the hip joints of children younger than age 3
- Can be unilateral or bilateral and affects the left hip more commonly than the right
- Three degrees of severity: dislocatable (hip positioned normally but manipulation can cause dislocation), subluxatable (femoral head rides on edge of acetabulum), or dislocated (femoral head totally outside acetabulum)

Causes
- Unknown
- Risk factors: breech delivery, elevated maternal relaxin, or large neonates or twins

Pathophysiologic changes

Unilateral dysplasia ➤	Limp
Hip rides above the acetabulum ➤	Uneven levels of the knees
Displacement of bones within the joint ➤	Joint structure damage; disrupted blood flow to the joint and ischemia

HIP DISPLACEMENT

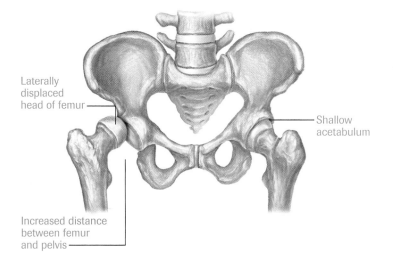

Laterally displaced head of femur

Shallow acetabulum

Increased distance between femur and pelvis

SIGNS OF DEVELOPMENTAL DYSPLASIA OF THE HIP

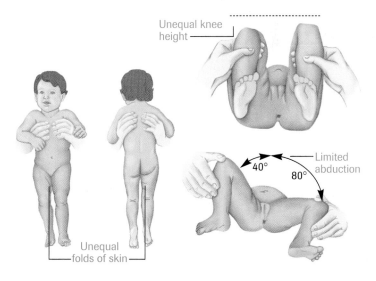

Unequal knee height

Unequal folds of skin

Limited abduction

40°

80°

Fractures

- Occur when a force exceeds the compressive or tensile strength of the bone
- Prognosis variable based on the extent of damage and the previous health and nutritional status of the patient

Causes

- Bone tumors
- Drugs that impair judgment or mobility
- Falls, motor vehicle accidents, sports
- Medications (such as corticosteroids) that cause iatrogenic osteoporosis
- Metabolic illness
- Young age

Pathophysiologic changes

Unnatural alignment ➤	Deformity, muscle spasms, limited range of motion (ROM)
Inflammatory response ➤	Swelling, tenderness, pain
Pinched or severed neurovascular structures from trauma or bone fragments ➤	Impaired sensation distal to the fracture site
Shifting bone fragments ➤	Limited ROM; crepitus sounds with movement

UNDERSTANDING COMMON FRACTURES

FRACTURE OF THE ELBOW

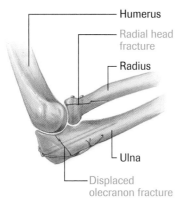

Humerus

Radial head fracture

Radius

Ulna

Displaced olecranon fracture

FRACTURE OF THE HAND AND WRIST

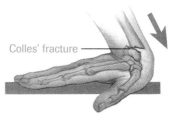

Colles' fracture

FRACTURES OF THE HIP

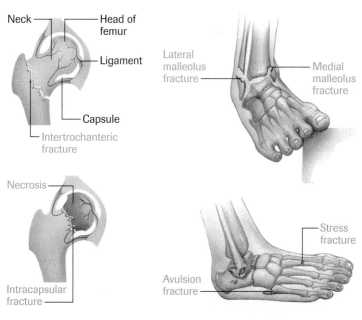

Neck

Head of femur

Ligament

Capsule

Intertrochanteric fracture

Necrosis

Intracapsular fracture

FRACTURES OF THE FOOT AND ANKLE

Lateral malleolus fracture

Medial malleolus fracture

Stress fracture

Avulsion fracture

Gout

- Metabolic disease marked by urate deposits that cause painfully arthritic joints
- Most commonly affects the foot
- Follows an intermittent course; good prognosis with treatment (unless it damages the renal tubules)

Causes
- Primary gout (possibly a genetic defect in purine metabolism)
- Secondary gout (certain drugs, diabetes mellitus, hypertension, obesity, renal disease, and sickle cell anemia)

Pathophysiologic changes

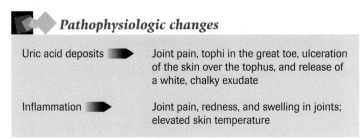

Uric acid deposits ➤	Joint pain, tophi in the great toe, ulceration of the skin over the tophus, and release of a white, chalky exudate
Inflammation ➤	Joint pain, redness, and swelling in joints; elevated skin temperature

GOUT OF THE KNEE

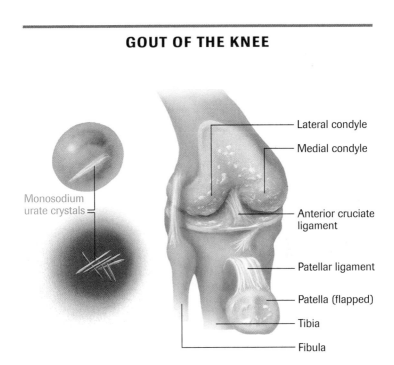

Monosodium urate crystals

Lateral condyle

Medial condyle

Anterior cruciate ligament

Patellar ligament

Patella (flapped)

Tibia

Fibula

GOUT OF THE FOOT

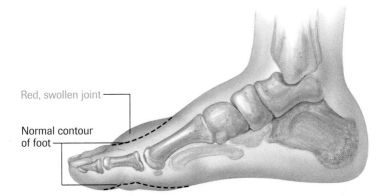

Red, swollen joint

Normal contour of foot

Muscular dystrophy

- Group of congenital disorders characterized by progressive symmetric wasting of skeletal muscles without sensory or neural defects
- Four main types: Duchenne's (or pseudohypertrophic), Becker's (or benign pseudohypertrophic), facioscapulohumeral (or Landouzy-Dejerine dystrophy), and limb-girdle

Causes

- Genetic mechanisms, typically causing an enzymatic or metabolic defect

Pathophysiologic changes

Inflammatory response ➤	Scarring and loss of muscle function
Progressive muscle wasting ➤	Mobility difficulties; poor balance; changes in physical appearance, such as a pendulous lip and absent nasolabial fold with facio-scapulohumeral dystrophy; limp; swaying
Connective muscle and fat replacing muscle tissue ➤	False impression of increased muscle mass, skeletal deformity, progressive immobility
Weakened cardiac and respiratory muscles ➤	Tachycardia, electrocardiographic abnormalities, pulmonary complications

MUSCLES AFFECTED IN DIFFERENT TYPES OF MUSCULAR DYSTROPHY

DUCHENNE'S

LIMB-GIRDLE

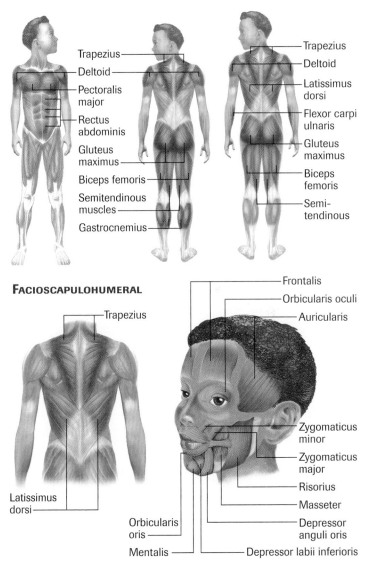

Duchenne's labels:
Trapezius
Deltoid
Pectoralis major
Rectus abdominis
Gluteus maximus
Biceps femoris
Semitendinous muscles
Gastrocnemius

Limb-girdle labels:
Trapezius
Deltoid
Latissimus dorsi
Flexor carpi ulnaris
Gluteus maximus
Biceps femoris
Semi-tendinous

FACIOSCAPULOHUMERAL

Trapezius
Latissimus dorsi

Frontalis
Orbicularis oculi
Auricularis
Zygomaticus minor
Zygomaticus major
Risorius
Masseter
Depressor anguli oris
Depressor labii inferioris
Orbicularis oris
Mentalis

Muscular dystrophy   231

Osteoarthritis

- Most common form of arthritis
- Chronic condition causing deterioration of joint cartilage and formation of reactive new bone at margins and subchondral areas of joints
- Usually affects weight-bearing joints (knees, feet, hips, lumbar vertebrae)

Causes

IDIOPATHIC OSTEOARTHRITIS
- Chemical factors (drugs that stimulate collagen-digesting enzymes in synovial membrane, such as steroids)
- Genetic factors (decreased collagen synthesis) and metabolic factors (endocrine disorders)
- Mechanical factors (repeated stress on joint)

SECONDARY OSTEOARTHRITIS
- Congenital deformity
- Obesity
- Trauma

Pathophysiologic changes

Degradation of cartilage, inflammation, and bone stress ➤	Deep, aching joint pain (usually relieved by rest); stiffness (in the morning and after exercise, usually relieved by rest)
Repeated inflammation ➤	Heberden's nodes (bony enlargements of distal interphalangeal joints)
Overcompensation of muscles supporting joints ➤	Altered gain from contractures
Pain and stiffness ➤	Decreased range of motion
Bone stress and altered bone growth ➤	Joint deformity

OSTEOARTHRITIS OF THE HAND, KNEE, AND HIP

HAND

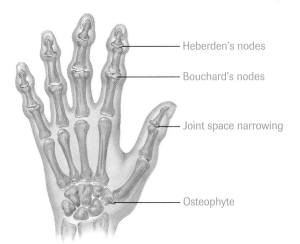

Heberden's nodes

Bouchard's nodes

Joint space narrowing

Osteophyte

RIGHT KNEE

Erosion of cartilage

Joint space narrowing

Osteophyte

HIP

Pelvis

Osteophyte

Erosion of cartilage

Erosion of bone

Osteomyelitis

■ Bone infection characterized by progressive inflammatory destruction after formation of new bone
■ Usually remains local but can spread to bone marrow, cortex, and periosteum
■ Acute osteomyelitis: usually blood-borne; commonly affecting rapidly growing children

Causes
■ Acute infection originating elsewhere in the body
■ Minor trauma

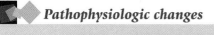

Pathophysiologic changes

Inflammation ➤	Sudden onset of pain in the affected bone; tenderness, heat, swelling, and restricted movement
Chronic infection ➤	Draining sinus tracts; widespread lesions

STAGES OF OSTEOMYELITIS

INITIAL INFECTION

FIRST STAGE

SECOND STAGE

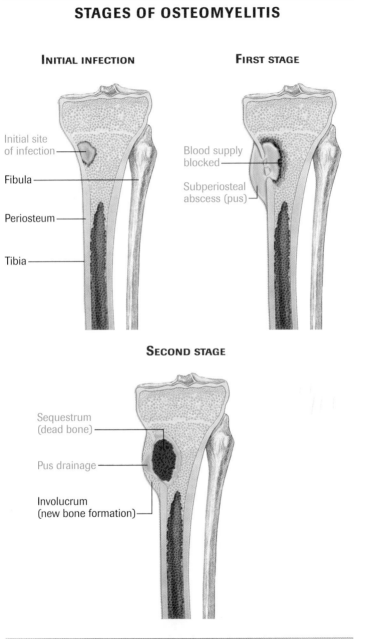

Initial site of infection

Fibula

Periosteum

Tibia

Blood supply blocked

Subperiosteal abscess (pus)

Sequestrum (dead bone)

Pus drainage

Involucrum (new bone formation)

Osteoporosis

- Metabolic bone disorder in which rate of bone resorption acceler- ates while rate of bone formation slows, causing loss of bone mass
- Loss of calcium and phosphate salts in affected bones, making them porous, brittle, and abnormally vulnerable to fractures
- May be classified as primary disease (commonly called *post- menopausal osteoporosis*) or secondary to other causes

Causes

- Unknown (in primary disease) but linked to many risk factors
- Medications (aluminum-containing antacids, anticonvulsants, corticosteroids)
- Osteogenesis imperfecta
- Prolonged therapy involving heparin or steroids
- Total immobility or disease of bone

Pathophysiologic changes

Weakened bones ▶	Loss of height; spinal deformities; sponta- neous wedge fractures, pathologic fractures of neck and femur, Colles' fractures of distal radius, vertebral collapse, and hip fractures
Fractures ▶	Pain

CALCIUM METABOLISM IN OSTEOPOROSIS

Normally, blood absorbs calcium from the digestive system and deposits it in the bones. In osteoporosis, blood levels of calcium are reduced. To maintain blood calcium levels as normal as possible, reabsorption from the bones increases.

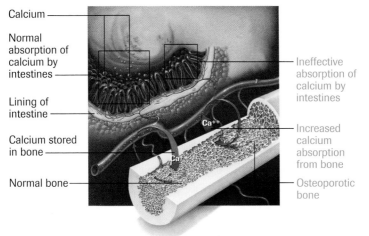

Calcium

Normal absorption of calcium by intestines

Lining of intestine

Calcium stored in bone

Normal bone

Ineffective absorption of calcium by intestines

Increased calcium absorption from bone

Osteoporotic bone

Bone formation and resorption

The organic portion of bone, called *osteoid,* acts as the matrix or framework for the mineral portion.

Bone cells called *osteoblasts* produce the osteoid matrix. The mineral portion, which consists of calcium and other minerals, hardens the osteoid matrix.

Large bone cells called *osteoclasts* reshape mature bone by resorbing the mineral and organic components. However, in osteoporosis, osteoblasts continue to produce bone but resorption by osteoclasts exceeds bone formation.

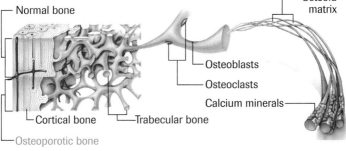

Osteoid matrix

Normal bone

Osteoblasts

Osteoclasts

Calcium minerals

Cortical bone

Trabecular bone

Osteoporotic bone

Scoliosis

- Lateral curvature of the thoracic, lumbar, or thoracolumbar spine
- Two types: functional (reversible deformity of the spinal column) or structural (fixed deformity of the spinal column)
- May be associated with kyphosis (humpback) or lordosis (swayback)

Causes

FUNCTIONAL

- Poor posture
- Uneven leg length

STRUCTURAL

- Congenital — wedge vertebrae, fused ribs or vertebrae, hemivertebrae
- Idiopathic — most common; appearing in a previously straight spine during the growing years; may be transmitted as an autosomal dominant or multifactorial trait
- Musculoskeletal or paralytic — asymmetric paralysis of trunk muscles due to polio, cerebral palsy, or muscular dystrophy

Pathophysiologic changes

Compensatory curve to maintain body balance ➡	One hip appearing higher than the other, uneven hemlines or pant legs, asymmetric gait, unequal shoulder heights, misalignment of the spinal vertebrae
Curvature greater than 40 degrees ➡	Back pain, pulmonary insufficiency, degenerative arthritis of the spine, vertebral disk disease, sciatica

NORMAL AND ABNORMAL CURVATURES OF THE SPINE

NORMAL

SCOLIOSIS

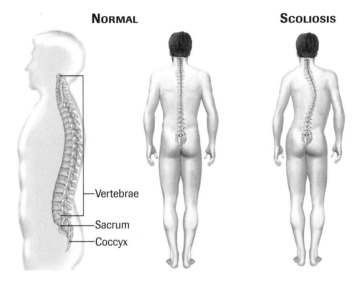

Vertebrae

Sacrum

Coccyx

Sprains

- Complete or incomplete tear of the supporting ligaments surrounding a joint when a joint forces beyond its normal range of motion
- May be accompanied by joint dislocations and fractures
- Ankle the most commonly sprained joint; finger, wrist, knee, and shoulder sprains also common

Causes
- Falls
- Motor vehicle accidents
- Sports injuries

Pathophysiologic changes

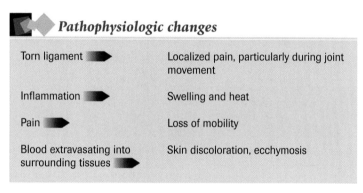

Torn ligament ➤	Localized pain, particularly during joint movement
Inflammation ➤	Swelling and heat
Pain ➤	Loss of mobility
Blood extravasating into surrounding tissues ➤	Skin discoloration, ecchymosis

THREE-LIGAMENT SPRAIN

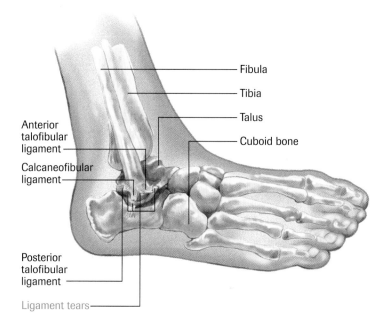

Fibula

Tibia

Talus

Cuboid bone

Anterior talofibular ligament

Calcaneofibular ligament

Posterior talofibular ligament

Ligament tears

Strains

- Injury to a muscle-tendon unit
- Sudden forceful contraction of a muscle under stretch that overloads its tensile strength, resulting in failure at the muscle-tendon junction
- Muscles that cross two joints most susceptible

Causes

- Degenerative changes in muscle-tendon units secondary to aging; anabolic steroid use
- Inadequate conditioning and stretching
- Sudden or unanticipated muscle contraction due to falling, sprinting, throwing, or other forceful activity

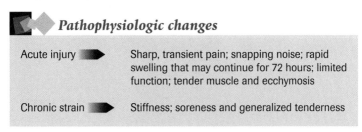

Pathophysiologic changes

Acute injury ➤	Sharp, transient pain; snapping noise; rapid swelling that may continue for 72 hours; limited function; tender muscle and ecchymosis
Chronic strain ➤	Stiffness; soreness and generalized tenderness

MUSCLE STRAIN

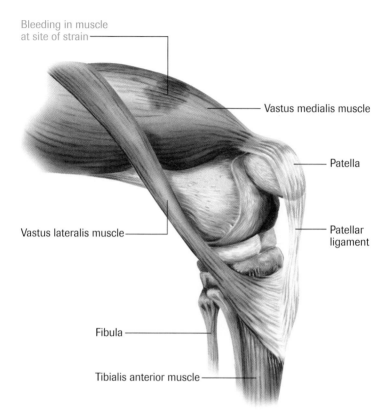

Bleeding in muscle at site of strain

Vastus medialis muscle

Patella

Vastus lateralis muscle

Patellar ligament

Fibula

Tibialis anterior muscle

Tendinitis

- Painful inflammation of tendons and tendon-muscle attachments to bone
- Occurs especially in the shoulder rotator cuff, Achilles tendon, or hamstring
- Osgood-Schlatter disease: common form of tendinitis, also known as *patellar tendinitis;* occurs in adolescence
- Achilles tendinitis: also known as *Sever's disease*

Causes
- Abnormal body development
- Hypermobility
- Other musculoskeletal disorders, such as rheumatic diseases and congenital defects
- Overuse, such as strain during sports activity
- Postural misalignment

Pathophysiologic changes

Inflammation ➡	Localized pain, restricted range of motion, swelling, crepitus
Calcium deposits in the tendon ➡	Proximal weakness; calcium erosion into the adjacent bursae

ELBOW TENDINITIS

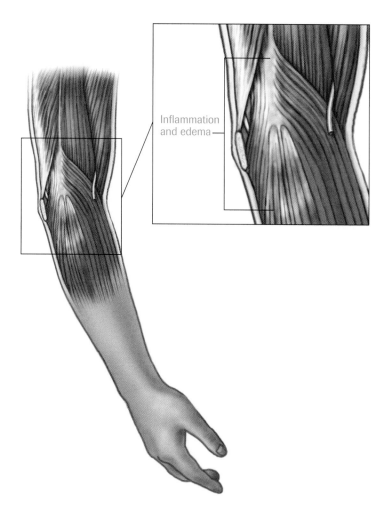

Inflammation and edema

6

Hematologic system

Acute leukemia

- Group of malignant disorders characterized by abnormal proliferation and maturation of lymphocytes and nonlymphocytic cells, leading to suppression of normal cells
- Acute lymphocytic leukemia: abnormal growth of lymphocytic precursors (lymphoblasts)
- Acute myelogenous leukemia: rapid accumulation of myeloid precursors (myeloblasts)

Causes
- Unknown
- Possible risk factors: exposure to chemicals and radiation, genetic predisposition, immunologic factors, predisposing disease

Pathophysiologic changes

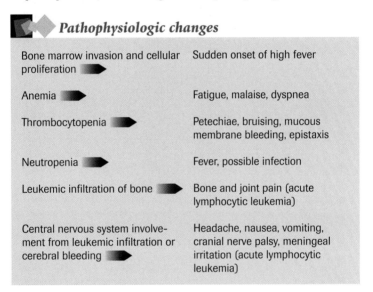

Bone marrow invasion and cellular proliferation ➡	Sudden onset of high fever
Anemia ➡	Fatigue, malaise, dyspnea
Thrombocytopenia ➡	Petechiae, bruising, mucous membrane bleeding, epistaxis
Neutropenia ➡	Fever, possible infection
Leukemic infiltration of bone ➡	Bone and joint pain (acute lymphocytic leukemia)
Central nervous system involvement from leukemic infiltration or cerebral bleeding ➡	Headache, nausea, vomiting, cranial nerve palsy, meningeal irritation (acute lymphocytic leukemia)

HISTOLOGIC FINDINGS OF ACUTE LYMPHOCYTIC LEUKEMIA

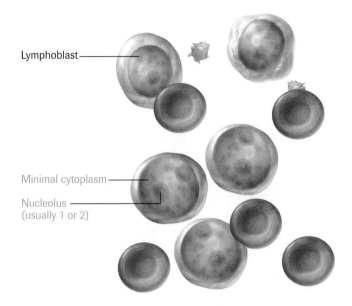

Lymphoblast

Minimal cytoplasm

Nucleolus
(usually 1 or 2)

Acute myelogenous leukemia

- Disease resulting from rapid accumulation of myeloid precursors (myeloblasts)
- Rapid onset and progression
- Leukemias most common malignancies in children; prognosis generally better in children than in adults

Causes
- Unknown
- Possible risk factors: exposure to chemicals and radiation, genetic predisposition, immunologic factors, predisposing disease

Pathophysiologic changes

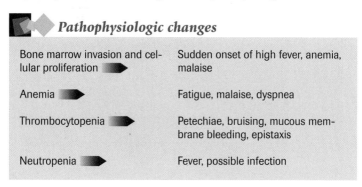

Bone marrow invasion and cellular proliferation ➤	Sudden onset of high fever, anemia, malaise
Anemia ➤	Fatigue, malaise, dyspnea
Thrombocytopenia ➤	Petechiae, bruising, mucous membrane bleeding, epistaxis
Neutropenia ➤	Fever, possible infection

HISTOLOGIC FINDINGS OF ACUTE MYELOGENOUS LEUKEMIA

Auer rod

Myeloblast

Large nucleus

Scant cytoplasm

Nucleoli
(usually 2 to 5)

Auer rod

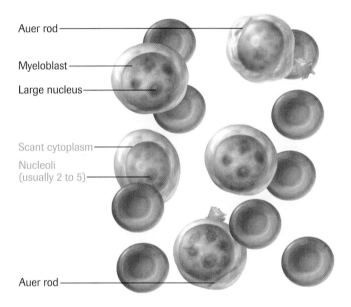

Anemia, aplastic

- Lower than normal levels of erythrocytes in the blood
- Usually develops when damaged or destroyed stem cells inhibit blood cell production
- Less commonly caused by damage to bone marrow microvasculature that inhibits cell growth and maturation
- Leads to pancytopenia (anemia, leukopenia, thrombocytopenia)

Causes

- Autoimmune reactions or other severe disease (hepatitis)
- Congenital
- Drugs (antibiotics, anticonvulsants)
- Radiation
- Toxic agents (benzene)

Pathophysiologic changes

Decreased red blood cell production ➡	Progressive weakness and fatigue, shortness of breath, headache, pallor and, ultimately, tachycardia and heart failure due to hypoxia and increased venous return
Thrombocytopenia ➡	Ecchymosis, petechiae, and hemorrhage, especially from the mucous membranes or into the retina or central nervous system
Neutropenia ➡	Infection, fever, oral and rectal ulcers, sore throat

PERIPHERAL BLOOD SMEAR
IN APLASTIC ANEMIA

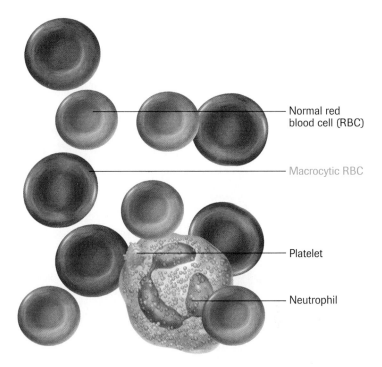

Normal red blood cell (RBC)

Macrocytic RBC

Platelet

Neutrophil

___ Anemia, iron deficiency ___

- Oxygen transport disorder characterized by deficiency in hemoglobin synthesis
- Most common in premenopausal women, infants (particularly premature and low birth weight), children, and adolescents (especially girls)
- Favorable prognosis following replacement therapy

Causes
- Blood loss from cancer, drug-induced GI bleeding, excessive blood sampling, heavy menses, peptic ulcer, sequestration, traumatic hemorrhage, varices
- Inadequate dietary intake of iron
- Intravascular hemolysis-induced hemoglobinuria, paroxysmal nocturnal hemoglobin
- Iron malabsorption
- Mechanical trauma to red blood cells
- Pregnancy

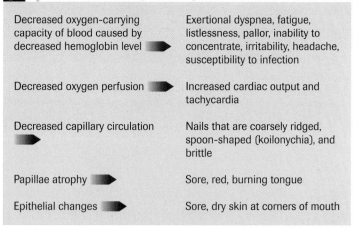

Pathophysiologic changes

Decreased oxygen-carrying capacity of blood caused by decreased hemoglobin level ▶	Exertional dyspnea, fatigue, listlessness, pallor, inability to concentrate, irritability, headache, susceptibility to infection
Decreased oxygen perfusion ▶	Increased cardiac output and tachycardia
Decreased capillary circulation ▶	Nails that are coarsely ridged, spoon-shaped (koilonychia), and brittle
Papillae atrophy ▶	Sore, red, burning tongue
Epithelial changes ▶	Sore, dry skin at corners of mouth

PERIPHERAL BLOOD SMEAR
IN IRON DEFICIENCY ANEMIA

Platelet

Cigar-shaped cells

Normal red blood cell (RBC)

Microcytic, hypochromic RBC

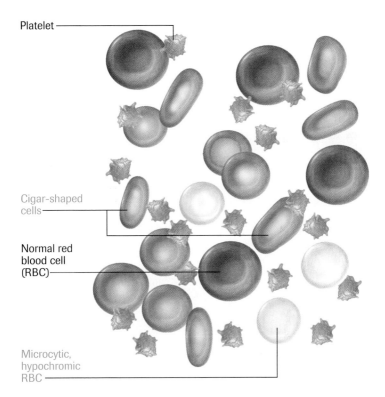

Anemia, pernicious

- Most common type of megaloblastic anemia
- Characterized by lack of intrinsic factor (needed to absorb vitamin B_{12}) and widespread red blood cell destruction
- Characteristic manifestations subsiding with treatment; some neurologic deficits possibly permanent

Causes
- Aging
- Genetic predisposition
- Immunologically related diseases
- Partial gastrectomy

Pathophysiologic changes

Tissue hypoxia ➤	Weakness, pale lips and gums
Atrophy of papillae ➤	Sore tongue
Interference with nerve impulse transmission ➤	Numbness and tingling in extremities; lack of coordination; ataxia; impaired fine finger movements; altered vision, taste, and hearing; loss of bowel and bladder control; impotence in males
Hemolysis-induced hyperbilirubinemia ➤	Faintly jaundiced sclera, pale to bright yellow skin
Gastric mucosal atrophy and decreased hydrochloric acid production ➤	Nausea, vomiting, anorexia, weight loss, flatulence, diarrhea, constipation
Compensatory increased cardiac output ➤	Palpitations, wide pulse pressure, dyspnea, orthopnea, tachycardia, premature beats, heart failure

PERIPHERAL BLOOD
SMEAR IN PERNICIOUS ANEMIA

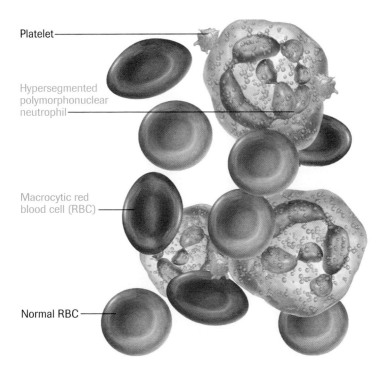

Platelet

Hypersegmented
polymorphonuclear
neutrophil

Macrocytic red
blood cell (RBC)

Normal RBC

Chronic lymphocytic leukemia

- Uncontrollable spread of small, abnormal lymphocytes in lymphoid tissue, blood, and bone marrow
- Slower onset and progression than acute leukemia

Causes
- Unknown
- Possible risk factors: exposure to chemicals and radiation, genetic predisposition, immunologic factors, predisposing disease

Pathophysiologic changes

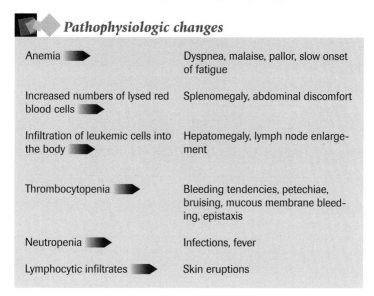

Anemia ▶	Dyspnea, malaise, pallor, slow onset of fatigue
Increased numbers of lysed red blood cells ▶	Splenomegaly, abdominal discomfort
Infiltration of leukemic cells into the body ▶	Hepatomegaly, lymph node enlargement
Thrombocytopenia ▶	Bleeding tendencies, petechiae, bruising, mucous membrane bleeding, epistaxis
Neutropenia ▶	Infections, fever
Lymphocytic infiltrates ▶	Skin eruptions

HISTOLOGIC FINDINGS
OF CHRONIC LYMPHOCYTIC LEUKEMIA

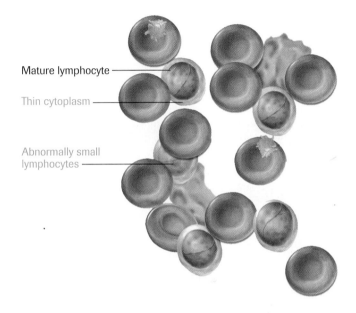

Mature lymphocyte

Thin cytoplasm

Abnormally small
lymphocytes

Chronic myeloid leukemia

- Abnormal overgrowth of granulocytic precursors (myeloblasts, promyelocytes, metamyelocytes, and myelocytes) in bone marrow, blood, and body tissues
- Proceeds in two distinct phases:
  - Insidious chronic phase: anemia and bleeding disorders
  - Blastic crisis or acute phase: rapid proliferation of myeloblasts, the most primitive granulocyte precursors

Causes
- Unknown
- Possible risk factors: exposure to chemicals and radiation, genetic predisposition, immunologic factors, predisposing disease

Pathophysiologic changes

Anemia ➤	Dyspnea, malaise, pallor, slow onset of fatigue
Thrombocytopenia ➤	Bleeding tendencies, petechiae, bruising, mucous membrane bleeding, epistaxis
Lymphadenopathy, splenomegaly, hepatomegaly ➤	Abdominal discomfort
Neutropenia ➤	Infections, fever
Lymphocytic infiltrates ➤	Skin eruptions

HISTOLOGIC FINDINGS
OF CHRONIC MYELOID LEUKEMIA

Neutrophil

Myeloblast

Increased
granulocytic line

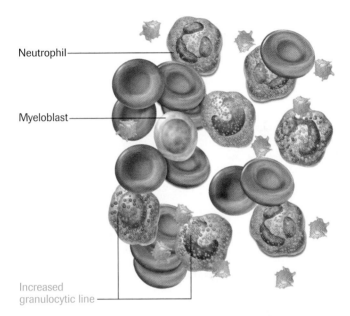

Disseminated — intravascular coagulation —

- Results in small blood vessel occlusion, organ necrosis, depletion of circulating clotting factors and platelets, activation of fibrinolytic system, and consequent severe hemorrhage
- Prognosis dependent on early detection and treatment, severity of hemorrhage, and treatment of underlying disease

Causes
- Infection
- Obstetric complications
- Necrotic disorders, such as brain tissue destruction, burns, liver necrosis, transplant rejection, and trauma
- Neoplastic disease
- Other causes: cardiac arrest, cirrhosis, fat embolism, giant hemangioma, heatstroke, incompatible blood transfusion, poisonous snakebite, purpura fulminans, severe venous thrombosis, shock, and surgery requiring cardiopulmonary bypass

Pathophysiologic changes

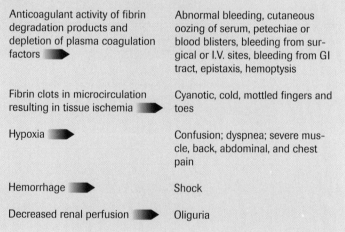

Anticoagulant activity of fibrin degradation products and depletion of plasma coagulation factors ➤	Abnormal bleeding, cutaneous oozing of serum, petechiae or blood blisters, bleeding from surgical or I.V. sites, bleeding from GI tract, epistaxis, hemoptysis
Fibrin clots in microcirculation resulting in tissue ischemia ➤	Cyanotic, cold, mottled fingers and toes
Hypoxia ➤	Confusion; dyspnea; severe muscle, back, abdominal, and chest pain
Hemorrhage ➤	Shock
Decreased renal perfusion ➤	Oliguria

NORMAL CLOTTING PROCESS

BLOOD VESSEL WALLS

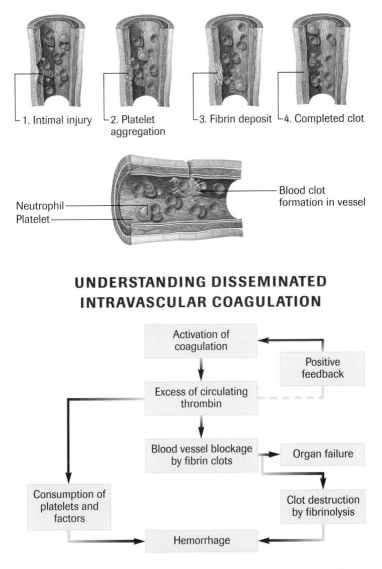

1. Intimal injury
2. Platelet aggregation
3. Fibrin deposit
4. Completed clot

Neutrophil
Platelet

Blood clot formation in vessel

UNDERSTANDING DISSEMINATED INTRAVASCULAR COAGULATION

Activation of coagulation

Positive feedback

Excess of circulating thrombin

Blood vessel blockage by fibrin clots → Organ failure

Consumption of platelets and factors

Clot destruction by fibrinolysis

Hemorrhage

Hemophilia

- X-linked recessive bleeding disorder resulting from deficiency of clotting factors
- Severity and prognosis of bleeding varyiable, depending on degree of deficiency or nonfunction and bleeding site
- Classification dependent on clotting factor involved
- Hemophilia A (classic hemophilia): deficiency of clotting factor VIII; affecting more than 80% of those with hemophilia
- Hemophilia B (Christmas disease): results from deficiency of factor IX; affecting about 15% of those with disorder
- Prevention of crippling deformities and prolonged life expectancy possible with proper treatment

Causes
- Chromosomal defects

Pathophysiologic changes

Lack of clotting factor ➤	Spontaneous bleeding (severe hemophilia); excessive or continued bleeding or bruising after minor trauma or surgery; large subcutaneous and deep intramuscular hematomas with mild trauma; pain, swelling, and tenderness from bleeding into joints, especially weight-bearing joints; internal bleeding commonly manifested as abdominal, chest, or flank pain; hematuria from bleeding into the kidney; hematemesis or tarry stools from bleeding into the GI tract

NORMAL CLOTTING AND CLOTTING IN HEMOPHILIA

NORMAL

HEMOPHILIA

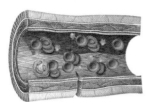
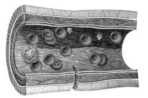

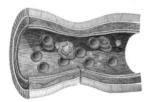
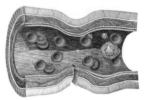

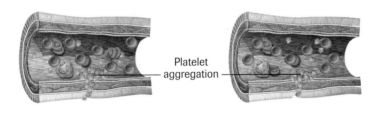

Platelet aggregation

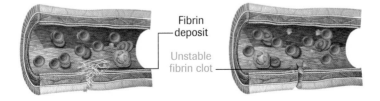

Fibrin deposit

Unstable fibrin clot

Hodgkin's disease

- Neoplastic disorder characterized by painless, progressive enlargement of lymph nodes, spleen, and other lymphoid tissue from proliferation of various blood cells
- Good prognosis with appropriate treatment (5-year survival rate of about 90%)

Causes
- Unknown
- Risk factors: age, environment, genetics, viral

Pathophysiologic changes

Proliferation of malignant cells ➤	Painless swelling of lymph nodes
Disease progression ➤	Fever, night sweats, fatigue, generalized pruritus
Lymph node enlargement in the chest ➤	Cough, chest pain, dyspnea

ANN ARBOR STAGING SYSTEM FOR HODGKIN'S DISEASE

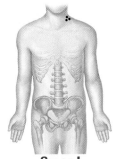

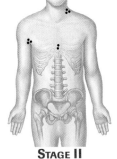

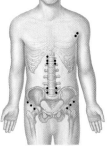

STAGE I
- Involvement of single lymph node region or
- Involvement of single extralymphatic site (stage I_E)

STAGE II
- Involvement of two or more lymph node regions on same side of diaphragm
- May include localized extralymphatic involvement on same side of diaphragm (stage II_E)

STAGE III
- Involvement of lymph node regions on both sides of diaphragm
- May include involvement of spleen (stage III_S), or localized extranodal disease (stage III_E)
- Hodgkin's disease stage III_1: disease limited to upper abdomen — spleen, splenic hilar, celiac, or portohepatic nodes
- Hodgkin's disease stage III_2: disease limited to lower abdomen — periaortic, pelvic, or inguinal nodes

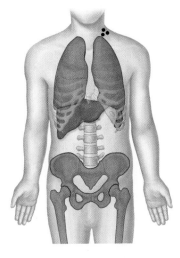

STAGE IV
- Diffuse extralymphatic disease (for example, in liver, bone marrow, lung, skin)

Multiple myeloma

- Disseminated malignant neoplasia of marrow plasma cells
- Infiltrates bone to produce osteolytic lesions throughout the skeleton
- Poor prognosis usually because diagnosis occurs after the disease has already infiltrated the vertebrae, pelvis, ribs, clavicles, and sternum

Causes

- Unknown

Pathophysiologic changes

Disease invasion of the bones of the body ➤	Severe, constant back pain; arthritis symptoms, including achiness, joint swelling, and tenderness; pathological fractures
Renal tubular damage from Bence Jones protein, hypercalcemia, and hyperuricemia ➤	Azotemia, pyelonephritis, renal failure
Altered bone marrow cell production ➤	Anemia, bleeding, infections
Vertebral compression ➤	Loss of height, peripheral neuropathies, thoracic deformities

BONE MARROW ASPIRATE
IN MULTIPLE MYELOMA

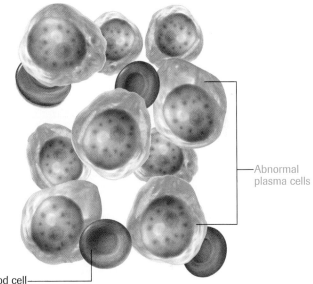

Abnormal plasma cells

Red blood cell

Non-Hodgkin's lymphoma

- Malignant lymphoma originating in lymph glands and other lymphoid tissue
- Three times more common than Hodgkin's disease
- Increasing incidence, especially in patients with autoimmune disorders or receiving immunosuppressant therapy

Causes
- Unknown

Pathophysiologic changes

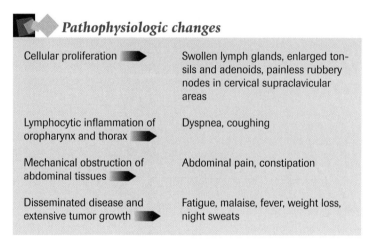

Cellular proliferation ➡	Swollen lymph glands, enlarged tonsils and adenoids, painless rubbery nodes in cervical supraclavicular areas
Lymphocytic inflammation of oropharynx and thorax ➡	Dyspnea, coughing
Mechanical obstruction of abdominal tissues ➡	Abdominal pain, constipation
Disseminated disease and extensive tumor growth ➡	Fatigue, malaise, fever, weight loss, night sweats

UNDERSTANDING THE LYMPHATIC SYSTEM

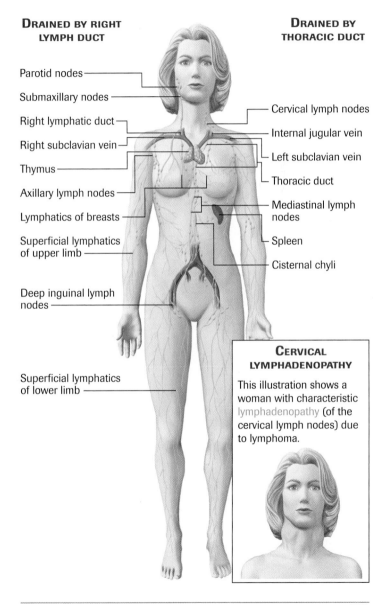

DRAINED BY RIGHT LYMPH DUCT

Parotid nodes

Submaxillary nodes

Right lymphatic duct

Right subclavian vein

Thymus

Axillary lymph nodes

Lymphatics of breasts

Superficial lymphatics of upper limb

Deep inguinal lymph nodes

Superficial lymphatics of lower limb

DRAINED BY THORACIC DUCT

Cervical lymph nodes

Internal jugular vein

Left subclavian vein

Thoracic duct

Mediastinal lymph nodes

Spleen

Cisternal chyli

CERVICAL LYMPHADENOPATHY

This illustration shows a woman with characteristic lymphadenopathy (of the cervical lymph nodes) due to lymphoma.

Polycythemia vera

- Chronic disorder characterized by increased red blood cell mass, erythrocytosis, leukocytosis, thrombocytosis, elevated hemoglobin level, and low or normal plasma volume
- Occurs most commonly among Jewish males of European descent
- Prognosis dependent on age at diagnosis, treatment, and complications

Causes

- Unknown but probably related to a clonal stem cell defect

Pathophysiologic changes

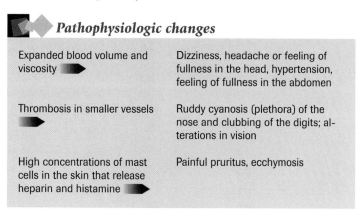

Expanded blood volume and viscosity ➤	Dizziness, headache or feeling of fullness in the head, hypertension, feeling of fullness in the abdomen
Thrombosis in smaller vessels ➤	Ruddy cyanosis (plethora) of the nose and clubbing of the digits; alterations in vision
High concentrations of mast cells in the skin that release heparin and histamine ➤	Painful pruritus, ecchymosis

PERIPHERAL BLOOD SMEAR
IN POLYCYTHEMIA

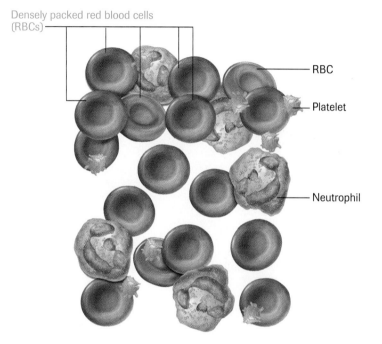

Densely packed red blood cells (RBCs)

RBC

Platelet

Neutrophil

Thalassemia

- Group of hereditary hemolytic anemias
- Results from defect in protein synthesis of hemoglobin
- Impairs red blood cell synthesis
- Most commonly occurs in people of Mediterranean ancestry
- Two forms of β-thalassemia (most common type): major and minor

Causes

- Heterozygous inheritance of the same gene (thalassemia minor)
- Homozygous inheritance of partially dominant autosomal gene (thalassemia major or intermedia)

Pathophysiologic changes

THALASSEMIA MAJOR

Mutation in beta globin chain of hemoglobin ➤	Underproduction of hemoglobin, severe anemia, pallor, bone abnormalities, fatigue, failure to thrive
Infection ➤	Fever
Erythroid hyperplasia and cortical bone thinning ➤	Deformed skull bones

THALASSEMIA MINOR

Mutation in one alpha globin chain of hemoglobin ➤	Mild anemia (carrier of genetic trait)

PERIPHERAL BLOOD SMEAR IN THALASSEMIA MAJOR

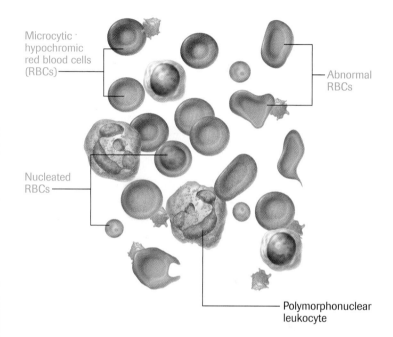

Microcytic hypochromic red blood cells (RBCs)

Abnormal RBCs

Nucleated RBCs

Polymorphonuclear leukocyte

7

Immune system

Acquired immunodeficiency syndrome

- Acquired through blood or body-fluid transmission of human immunodeficiency virus (HIV)
- Characterized by gradual destruction of cell-mediated (T-cell) immunity and autoimmunity, causing susceptibility to opportunistic infections, cancer, and other abnormalities
- Diagnosis based on HIV status and presence of fewer than 200 CD4+ T cells per cubic millimeter of blood

Cause
- Contact with HIV-infected blood or body fluids (HIV-1 or HIV-2)

Pathophysiologic changes

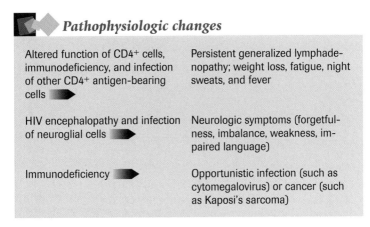

Altered function of CD4+ cells, immunodeficiency, and infection of other CD4+ antigen-bearing cells ➤	Persistent generalized lymphadenopathy; weight loss, fatigue, night sweats, and fever
HIV encephalopathy and infection of neuroglial cells ➤	Neurologic symptoms (forgetfulness, imbalance, weakness, impaired language)
Immunodeficiency ➤	Opportunistic infection (such as cytomegalovirus) or cancer (such as Kaposi's sarcoma)

MANIFESTATIONS OF HIV INFECTION AND AIDS

SYMPTOMS OF HIV INFECTION

AIDS-RELATED ILLNESSES AND OPPORTUNISTIC INFECTIONS (OIs)

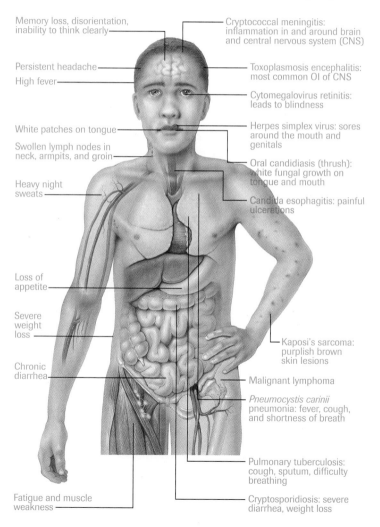

Memory loss, disorientation, inability to think clearly

Persistent headache

High fever

White patches on tongue

Swollen lymph nodes in neck, armpits, and groin

Heavy night sweats

Loss of appetite

Severe weight loss

Chronic diarrhea

Fatigue and muscle weakness

Cryptococcal meningitis: inflammation in and around brain and central nervous system (CNS)

Toxoplasmosis encephalitis: most common OI of CNS

Cytomegalovirus retinitis: leads to blindness

Herpes simplex virus: sores around the mouth and genitals

Oral candidiasis (thrush): white fungal growth on tongue and mouth

Candida esophagitis: painful ulcerations

Kaposi's sarcoma: purplish brown skin lesions

Malignant lymphoma

Pneumocystis carinii pneumonia: fever, cough, and shortness of breath

Pulmonary tuberculosis: cough, sputum, difficulty breathing

Cryptosporidiosis: severe diarrhea, weight loss

Acquired immunodeficiency syndrome   279

Allergic rhinitis

- Reaction to airborne (inhaled) allergens
- Depending on the allergen, may be seasonal or a year-round condition
- Most common atopic allergic reaction, affecting more than 20 million U.S. residents

Cause

- Immunoglobulin E–mediated type I hypersensitivity response to an environmental antigen (allergen) in a genetically susceptible person

Pathophysiologic changes

Release of histamine by the mast cells ➤	Paroxysmal sneezing; profuse watery rhinorrhea; pruritus of nose and eyes; red, edematous eyelids and conjunctivae; excessive lacrimation; increased mucus secretion in the nasal cavity and airways
Tightening of the smooth muscles in the airways ➤	Nasal obstruction or congestion; pale, cyanotic, edematous nasal mucosa; itching in the throat; wheezing
Dilation of small blood vessels ➤	Headache or sinus pain

REACTION TO ALLERGEN EXPOSURE

PRIMARY EXPOSURE

- Allergen
- B cell
- T cell
- Immunoglobulin (Ig) E antibodies attached to mast cell
- Blood vessel
- Mast cells

REEXPOSURE

- Mast cell
- Allergen
- IgE antibodies
- Histamine and other mediators

Anaphylaxis

- Acute, potentially life-threatening type I (immediate) hypersensitivity reaction marked by sudden onset of rapidly progressive urticaria (vascular swelling in skin accompanied by itching) and respiratory distress
- Occurs within minutes but can occur up to 1 hour after reexposure to antigen

Cause

- Ingestion of (or systemic exposure to) sensitizing drugs or other substances, such as antibiotics or other drugs, diagnostic chemicals, food proteins, insect venom, serums, and sulfite-containing food additives

Pathophysiologic changes

Histamine, serotonin, and leukotrienes release ➤	Nasal congestion, itchy and watery eyes, flushing, weakness, and anxiety
Eosinophil chemotactic factor of anaphylaxis (ECF-A) release ➤	Swelling and wheals
Endothelial destruction and fluid leak into alveoli and airways ➤	Edema of upper respiratory tract and respiratory distress
Increased vascular permeability and subsequent decrease in peripheral resistance and leakage of plasma fluids ➤	Vascular collapse; shock, confusion, tachycardia, and hypotension
Heparin and mediator-neutralizing substance release ➤	Hemorrhage, disseminated intravascular coagulation, and cardiac arrest

DEVELOPMENT OF ANAPHYLAXIS

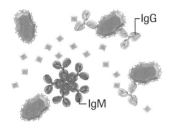

1. Response to antigen
Immunoglobulins (Ig) M and G recognize and bind the antigen.

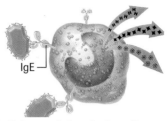

2. Release of chemical mediators
Activated IgE on basophils promotes the release of mediators: histamine, serotonin, and leukotrienes.

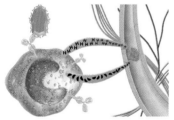

3. Intensified response
Mast cells release more histamine and ECF-A.

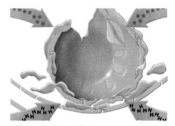

4. Respiratory distress
In the lungs, histamine causes endothelial cell destruction and fluid to leak into alveoli.

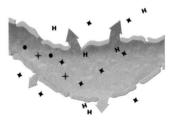

5. Deterioration
Meanwhile, mediators increase vascular permeability, causing fluid to leak from the vessels.

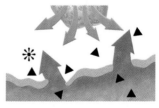

6. Failure of compensatory mechanisms
Endothelial cell damage causes basophils and mast cells to release heparin and mediator-neutralizing substances. However, anaphylaxis is now irreversible.

KEY

Complement cascade	▦	Serotonin	✖	Prostaglandins	✛	Bradykinin ●
Histamine	H	Leukotrienes	✳	ECF-A	◀	Heparin ▲

Ankylosing spondylitis

- Chronic, usually progressive inflammatory bone disease
- Primarily affects the sacroiliac, apophyseal, and costovertebral joints, along with adjacent soft tissue
- Well recognized in men but commonly overlooked or missed in women

Cause
- Unknown

Pathophysiologic changes

Collagen forms fibrous scar tissue that eventually calcifies and ossifies ➤	Fusion of the spine and peripheral joints; loss of flexibility; kyphosis, stiffness, and limited lumbar spine motion; hip deformity and limited range of motion; peripheral arthritis in shoulders, hips, and knees; pain and limited expansion of the chest wall; intermittent lower back pain that's most severe in the morning
Inflammatory processes ➤	Warmth, swelling, or tenderness of affected joints; mild fatigue; fever; anorexia; weight loss

SPINAL FUSION IN ANKYLOSING SPONDYLITIS

Lateral View

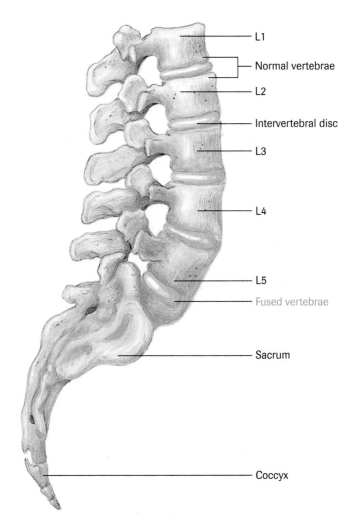

L1

Normal vertebrae

L2

Intervertebral disc

L3

L4

L5

Fused vertebrae

Sacrum

Coccyx

Rheumatoid arthritis

■ Chronic, systemic inflammatory disease that primarily attacks peripheral joints and surrounding muscles, tendons, ligaments, and blood vessels

■ Characterized by partial remissions and unpredictable exacerbations

Cause
■ Unknown

Pathophysiologic changes

Initial inflammatory reactions before inflammation of synovium ➤	Fatigue, malaise, anorexia and weight loss, persistent low-grade fever, lymphadenopathy, and vague articular symptoms
Prostaglandin release; inflammation and destruction of synovium ➤	Specific localized, bilateral, and symmetric articular symptoms; stiffening of affected joints after inactivity (especially on arising in the morning); spindle-shaped fingers; joint pain and tenderness; feeling of warmth at joint; rheumatoid nodules
Swelling and loss of joint space ➤	Flexion deformities or hyperextension of metacarpophalangeal joints; subluxation of the wrist; stretching of tendons, pulling fingers to ulnar side; characteristic swan-neck or boutonniere deformity
Infiltration of nerve fibers ➤	Peripheral neuropathy

THE EFFECTS OF RHEUMATOID ARTHRITIS ON CERTAIN JOINTS

KNEE

Erosion of cartilage

Erosion of bone

Pannus covering synovial membrane

HAND AND WRIST

Joint space narrowing

Joint capsule

Pannus

Swelling

Erosion of bone

Erosion

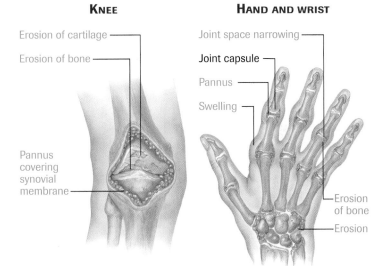

HIP

Erosion of cartilage

Pannus

Redness around joint

Erosion of bone

Femur

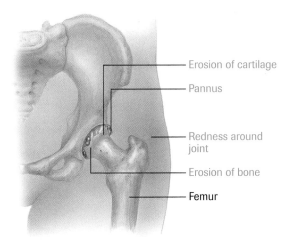

Scleroderma

- Autoimmune connective tissue disease
- Characterized by inflammatory, degenerative, and fibrotic changes in skin, blood vessels, synovial membranes, skeletal muscles, and internal organs
- May be localized (skin, musculoskeletal system) or generalized (skin, musculoskeletal system, internal organs)

Cause
- Unknown

Pathophysiologic changes

Excess collagen deposited in skin ➤	Skin changes: becoming hard and thick; ulcers or sores on fingers; loss of hair over affected area; change in color; swelling and puffiness in fingers and toes; shiny skin; disappearance of skin creases
Damage to small blood vessels ➤	Raynaud's phenomenon
Calcium deposits ➤	Calcinosis
Excess collagen in joint and muscles ➤	Arthritis and muscle weakness
Loss of lower esophageal sphincter function ➤	Frequent reflux, heartburn, dysphagia, and bloating after meals
Scarring of organs or thickening of blood vessels ➤	Heart or kidney failure, interstitial lung disease, and pulmonary hypertension

SCLERODACTYLY

Thin, shiny skin on fingers —

Flexed, stiff fingers —

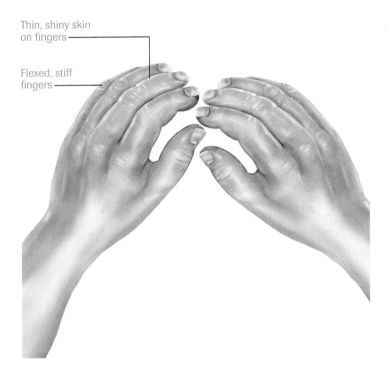

Systemic lupus erythematosus

- Chronic, inflammatory, autoimmune connective tissue disease
- Affects multiple organ systems
- Characterized by recurring remissions and exacerbations

Cause
- Unknown

Pathophysiologic changes

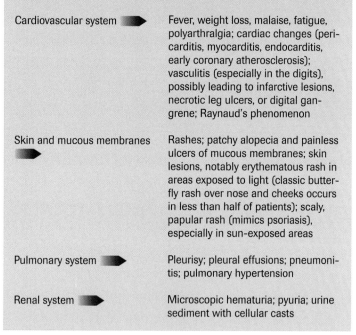

Tissue injury, inflammation, and necrosis from invasion by immune complexes in:

Cardiovascular system	Fever, weight loss, malaise, fatigue, polyarthralgia; cardiac changes (pericarditis, myocarditis, endocarditis, early coronary atherosclerosis); vasculitis (especially in the digits), possibly leading to infarctive lesions, necrotic leg ulcers, or digital gangrene; Raynaud's phenomenon
Skin and mucous membranes	Rashes; patchy alopecia and painless ulcers of mucous membranes; skin lesions, notably erythematous rash in areas exposed to light (classic butterfly rash over nose and cheeks occurs in less than half of patients); scaly, papular rash (mimics psoriasis), especially in sun-exposed areas
Pulmonary system	Pleurisy; pleural effusions; pneumonitis; pulmonary hypertension
Renal system	Microscopic hematuria; pyuria; urine sediment with cellular casts

THE EFFECTS OF SYSTEMIC LUPUS ERYTHEMATOSUS

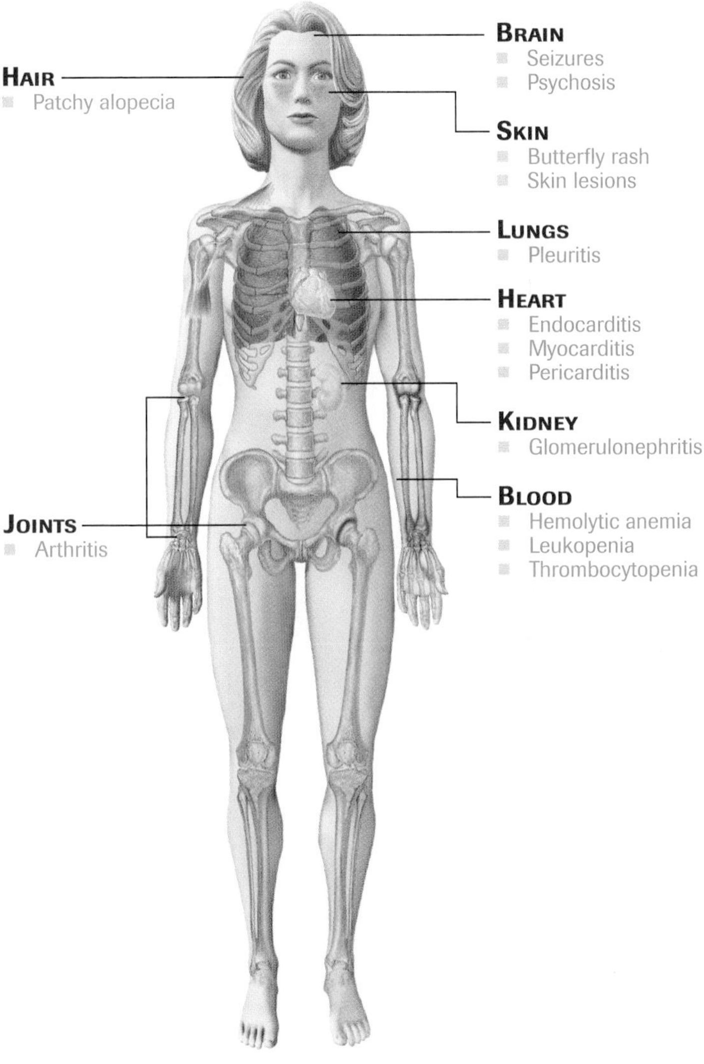

HAIR
- Patchy alopecia

BRAIN
- Seizures
- Psychosis

SKIN
- Butterfly rash
- Skin lesions

LUNGS
- Pleuritis

HEART
- Endocarditis
- Myocarditis
- Pericarditis

KIDNEY
- Glomerulonephritis

BLOOD
- Hemolytic anemia
- Leukopenia
- Thrombocytopenia

JOINTS
- Arthritis

8

*Endocrine
system*

Adrenal hypofunction

- Primary hypofunction (Addison's disease) that originates with the adrenal gland: characterized by decreased secretion of mineralocorticoids, glucocorticoids, and androgens and by destruction of the adrenal cortex
- Secondary hypofunction: characterized by decreased glucocorticoid secretion and unaffected aldosterone secretion

Causes

PRIMARY ADRENAL HYPOFUNCTION
- Autoimmune process
- Bilateral adrenalectomy
- Idiopathic atrophy of adrenal glands
- Neoplasms, tuberculosis, or other infections

SECONDARY ADRENAL HYPOFUNCTION
- Abrupt withdrawal of long-term corticosteroid therapy
- Hypopituitarism
- Removal of corticotropin-secreting tumor

Pathophysiologic changes

PRIMARY ADRENAL HYPOFUNCTION

Mineralocorticoid or glucocorticoid deficiency ➡	Weakness and fatigue; weight loss, nausea, vomiting, and anorexia; decreased tolerance for minor stress; cardiovascular abnormalities; craving for salty foods
Decreased cortisol levels and simultaneous secretion of excessive corticotropin and melanocyte-stimulating hormone ➡	Conspicuous bronze skin coloring, darkening of scars, areas of vitiligo, increased pigmentation of mucous membranes
Decreased gluconeogenesis ➡	Fasting hypoglycemia

SECONDARY ADRENAL HYPOFUNCTION
Signs and symptoms similar to those of primary hypofunction, but without hyperpigmentation

Acute adrenal crisis ➡	Profound weakness and fatigue, nausea and vomiting, dehydration, hypotension, high fever followed by hypothermia

ADRENAL HORMONE SECRETION

ADRENAL HORMONES

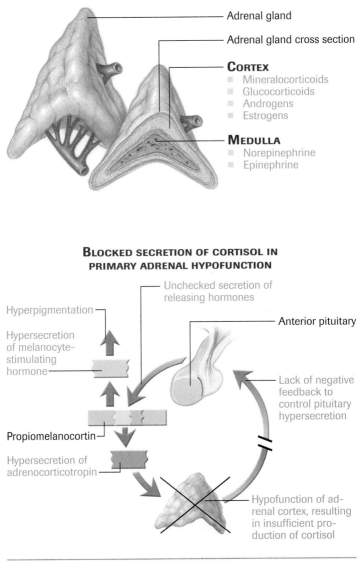

Adrenal gland

Adrenal gland cross section

CORTEX
- Mineralocorticoids
- Glucocorticoids
- Androgens
- Estrogens

MEDULLA
- Norepinephrine
- Epinephrine

BLOCKED SECRETION OF CORTISOL IN PRIMARY ADRENAL HYPOFUNCTION

Unchecked secretion of releasing hormones

Hyperpigmentation

Hypersecretion of melanocyte-stimulating hormone

Propiomelanocortin

Hypersecretion of adrenocorticotropin

Anterior pituitary

Lack of negative feedback to control pituitary hypersecretion

Hypofunction of adrenal cortex, resulting in insufficient production of cortisol

Cushing's syndrome

- Cluster of clinical abnormalities caused by excessive adrenocortical hormones
- Cushing's disease (pituitary corticotropin excess): accounts for about 80% of endogenous cases

Causes
- Ectopic corticotropin secretion by a tumor outside the pituitary gland
- Excessive or prolonged use of glucocorticoids
- Excess of anterior pituitary hormone (corticotropin)

Pathophysiologic changes

Cortisol-induced insulin resistance and increased gluconeogenesis in the liver ➧	Diabetes mellitus, decreased glucose tolerance, hyperglycemia, and glucosuria
Increased androgen production ➧	Mild virilism, hirsutism, clinical hypertrophy, and amenorrhea or oligomenorrhea; sexual dysfunction
Hypokalemia ➧	Muscle weakness
Bone porosity and disease ➧	Pathologic fractures
Decreased collagen and weakened tissue ➧	Striae; facial plethora; acne; fat pads above clavicles, over upper back, on face, and throughout trunk with slender arms and legs; little or no scar formation; poor wound healing; spontaneous ecchymosis; hyperpigmentation
Increased gastric secretion and pepsin production ➧	Peptic ulcer; abdominal pain; increased appetite; weight gain
Sodium and fluid retention ➧	Hypertension; heart failure; left ventricular hypertrophy
Protein loss ➧	Capillary weakness, bleeding, and ecchymosis
Altered neurotransmission ➧	Irritability and emotional lability

MANIFESTATIONS OF CUSHING'S SYNDROME

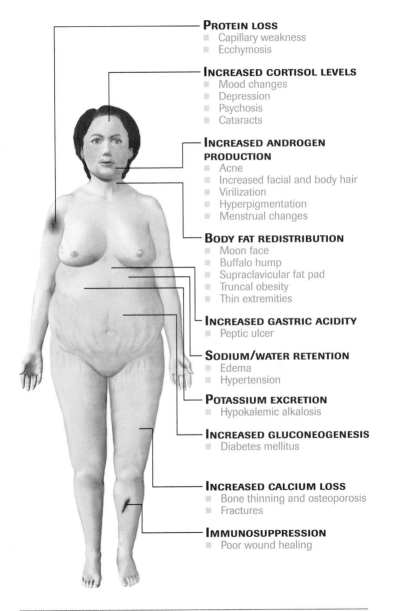

PROTEIN LOSS
- Capillary weakness
- Ecchymosis

INCREASED CORTISOL LEVELS
- Mood changes
- Depression
- Psychosis
- Cataracts

INCREASED ANDROGEN PRODUCTION
- Acne
- Increased facial and body hair
- Virilization
- Hyperpigmentation
- Menstrual changes

BODY FAT REDISTRIBUTION
- Moon face
- Buffalo hump
- Supraclavicular fat pad
- Truncal obesity
- Thin extremities

INCREASED GASTRIC ACIDITY
- Peptic ulcer

SODIUM/WATER RETENTION
- Edema
- Hypertension

POTASSIUM EXCRETION
- Hypokalemic alkalosis

INCREASED GLUCONEOGENESIS
- Diabetes mellitus

INCREASED CALCIUM LOSS
- Bone thinning and osteoporosis
- Fractures

IMMUNOSUPPRESSION
- Poor wound healing

Diabetes insipidus

- Results from a deficiency of circulating vasopressin (antidiuretic hormone, or ADH) or from renal resistance to this hormone
- Characterized by excessive fluid intake and hypotonic polyuria
- Three forms: nephrogenic, neurogenic, and psychogenic

Causes

- Nephrogenic — end-stage renal failure or X-linked recessive trait
- Neurogenic — cranial trauma, hypothalamic or pituitary tumor, stroke, or surgery
- Psychogenic — primary polydipsia or sarcoidosis
- Transient diabetes insipidus — certain drugs (alcohol, lithium, or phenytoin)

Pathophysiologic changes

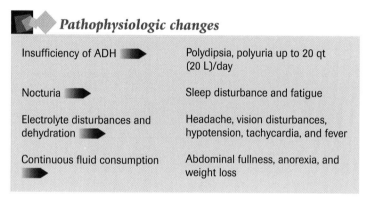

Insufficiency of ADH ➤	Polydipsia, polyuria up to 20 qt (20 L)/day
Nocturia ➤	Sleep disturbance and fatigue
Electrolyte disturbances and dehydration ➤	Headache, vision disturbances, hypotension, tachycardia, and fever
Continuous fluid consumption ➤	Abdominal fullness, anorexia, and weight loss

MECHANISM OF ADH DEFICIENCY

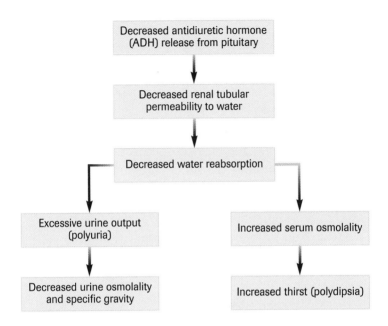

Diabetes mellitus

- Chronic disorder of carbohydrate metabolism with subsequent alteration of protein and fat metabolism
- Characterized by hyperglycemia that results from lack of insulin (type 1), lack of insulin effect (type 2), or both

Causes

TYPE 1 DIABETES

- Autoimmune process triggered by viral or environmental factors
- Idiopathic (no evidence of autoimmune process)

TYPE 2 DIABETES

- Beta cell exhaustion due to lifestyle habits or hereditary factors

Pathophysiologic changes

High serum osmolality caused by high serum glucose levels ➡	Polyuria and polydipsia
Depleted cellular storage of carbohydrates, fat, and protein ➡	Polyphagia
Prevention of normal metabolism of carbohydrates, fat, and protein caused by impaired or absent insulin function ➡	Weight loss
Low intracellular glucose levels ➡	Headache, fatigue, lethargy, and reduced energy level
Electrolyte imbalances ➡	Muscle cramps, irritability, and emotional lability
Glucose-induced swelling ➡	Vision changes
Neural tissue damage ➡	Numbness and tingling
Dehydration, electrolyte imbalances, and autonomic neuropathy ➡	Abdominal discomfort and pain; nausea, diarrhea, or constipation
Hyperglycemia ➡	Slowly healing skin infections or wounds, skin itching, vaginal pruritus and vulvovaginitis

TYPE 1 AND TYPE 2 DIABETES MELLITUS

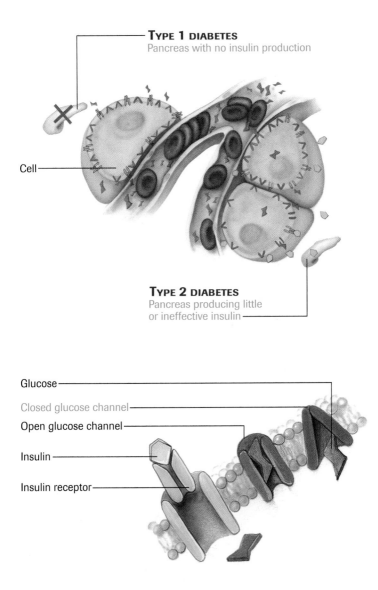

TYPE 1 DIABETES
Pancreas with no insulin production

Cell

TYPE 2 DIABETES
Pancreas producing little
or ineffective insulin

Glucose

Closed glucose channel

Open glucose channel

Insulin

Insulin receptor

Hyperthyroidism

- Metabolic imbalance that results from overproduction of thyroid hormone; also called *thyrotoxicosis*
- Graves' disease: increases thyroxine production, enlarges thyroid gland (goiter), and causes multiple system changes
- Thyroid storm: a medical emergency that produces life-threatening cardiac, hepatic, or renal consequences

Causes

- Autoimmune disease (Graves' disease)
- Genetic factors
- Increased thyroid-stimulating hormone secretions
- Thyroid adenomas
- Toxic multinodular goiter

Pathophysiologic changes

HYPERTHYROIDISM

Increased amounts of thyroid hormone ➡	Enlarged thyroid (goiter), excitability or nervousness, heat intolerance and sweating, weight loss (despite increased appetite), frequent bowel movements, palpitations, hypertension
Cytokine-mediated activation of orbital tissue fibroblasts ➡	Exophthalmos
Accelerated cerebral function ➡	Difficulty concentrating
Increased activity in spinal cord area that controls muscle tone ➡	Fine tremor, shaky handwriting, and clumsiness

THYROID STORM

Increased catecholamine response and hyperthyroid state ➡	High fever, tachycardia, pulmonary edema, hypertension, shock, tremors, emotional lability, extreme irritability, confusion, delirium, psychosis, apathy, stupor, diarrhea, abdominal pain, nausea, vomiting, jaundice, hyperglycemia, and coma

THYROID GLAND AND ITS HORMONES

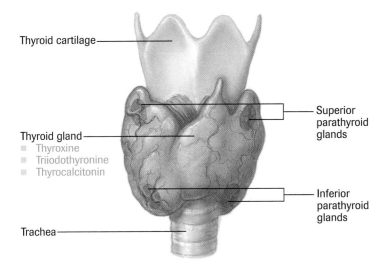

Thyroid cartilage

Thyroid gland
- Thyroxine
- Triiodothyronine
- Thyrocalcitonin

Trachea

Superior parathyroid glands

Inferior parathyroid glands

HISTOLOGIC CHANGES IN GRAVES' DISEASE

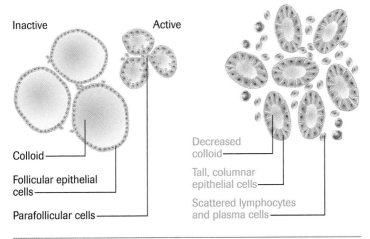

NORMAL

GRAVES' DISEASE

Inactive

Active

Colloid

Follicular epithelial cells

Parafollicular cells

Decreased colloid

Tall, columnar epithelial cells

Scattered lymphocytes and plasma cells

Hypothyroidism, adult

- Results from hypothalamic, pituitary, or thyroid insufficiency or resistance to thyroid hormone
- May lead to life-threatening myxedema coma

Causes

- Autoimmune disease (Hashimoto's thyroiditis)
- Malfunction of the pituitary gland
- Overuse of antithyroid drugs
- Radiation therapy (particularly with iodine 131)
- Thyroidectomy

Pathophysiologic changes

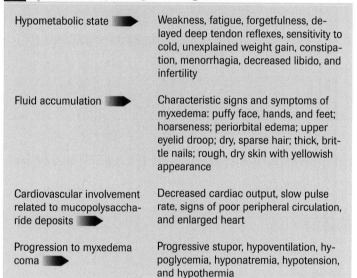

Hypometabolic state ▶	Weakness, fatigue, forgetfulness, delayed deep tendon reflexes, sensitivity to cold, unexplained weight gain, constipation, menorrhagia, decreased libido, and infertility
Fluid accumulation ▶	Characteristic signs and symptoms of myxedema: puffy face, hands, and feet; hoarseness; periorbital edema; upper eyelid droop; dry, sparse hair; thick, brittle nails; rough, dry skin with yellowish appearance
Cardiovascular involvement related to mucopolysaccharide deposits ▶	Decreased cardiac output, slow pulse rate, signs of poor peripheral circulation, and enlarged heart
Progression to myxedema coma ▶	Progressive stupor, hypoventilation, hypoglycemia, hyponatremia, hypotension, and hypothermia

HISTOLOGIC CHANGES IN HASHIMOTO'S THYROIDITIS

NORMAL

HASHIMOTO'S THYROIDITIS

Inactive   Active

Lymphocytes and
plasma cells

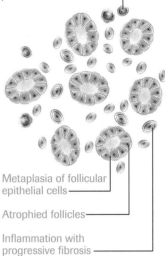

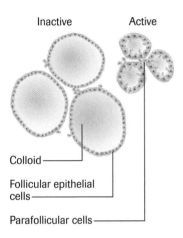

Colloid

Follicular epithelial
cells

Parafollicular cells

Metaplasia of follicular
epithelial cells

Atrophied follicles

Inflammation with
progressive fibrosis

Metabolic syndrome

- Characterized by obesity, high blood pressure, high blood glucose, and an abnormal cholesterol profile
- Increased risk of developing coronary heart disease, stroke, and diabetes

Cause
- Insulin resistance

Pathophysiologic changes

Increase in circulating insulin ▶	High glucose levels, hyperinsulinemia, and obesity
Vascular hypertrophy and remodeling ▶	Increased cholesterol and triglyceride levels, increased serum uric acid, increased platelet adhesion, increased response to angiotensin II, and decreased amounts of nitric oxide
Hormonal imbalances ▶	Irregular or absent menstrual periods, infertility, acne, hirsutism, alopecia

METABOLIC SYNDROME

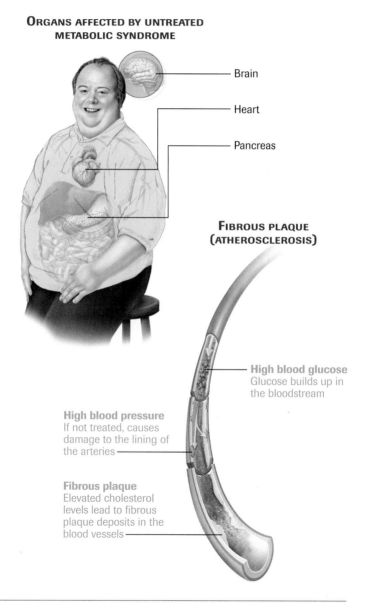

ORGANS AFFECTED BY UNTREATED METABOLIC SYNDROME

Brain

Heart

Pancreas

FIBROUS PLAQUE (ATHEROSCLEROSIS)

High blood glucose
Glucose builds up in the bloodstream

High blood pressure
If not treated, causes damage to the lining of the arteries

Fibrous plaque
Elevated cholesterol levels lead to fibrous plaque deposits in the blood vessels

Syndrome of inappropriate antidiuretic hormone

- Potentially life-threatening condition that disturbs fluid and electrolyte balance
- Results when excessive antidiuretic hormone (ADH) secretion is triggered by stimuli other than increased extracellular fluid osmolarity and decreased extracellular fluid volume; reflected by hypotension

Causes
- Central nervous system or respiratory system disorders
- Drugs that either increase ADH production or potentiate ADH action
- Neoplastic diseases
- Oat cell carcinoma of the lung
- Other conditions: acquired immunodeficiency syndrome, myxedema, pain, physiologic stress, psychosis

Pathophysiologic changes

Hyponatremia and electrolyte imbalances ➡	Thirst, anorexia, fatigue, and lethargy (first signs), followed by vomiting and intestinal cramping; weight gain, edema, water retention, and decreased urine output; neurologic changes (restlessness, confusion, headache, irritability, decreasing reflexes, and seizures); decreased deep tendon reflexes; and coma

WHAT HAPPENS IN SIADH

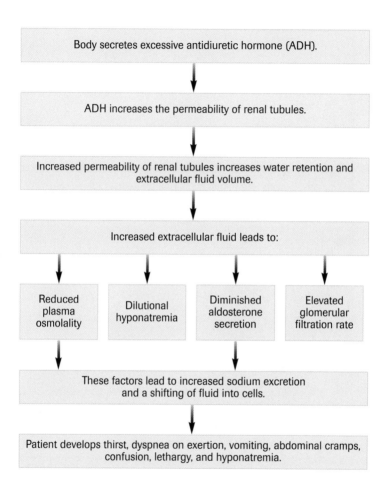

Body secretes excessive antidiuretic hormone (ADH).

↓

ADH increases the permeability of renal tubules.

↓

Increased permeability of renal tubules increases water retention and extracellular fluid volume.

↓

Increased extracellular fluid leads to:

↓

| Reduced plasma osmolality | Dilutional hyponatremia | Diminished aldosterone secretion | Elevated glomerular filtration rate |

↓

These factors lead to increased sodium excretion and a shifting of fluid into cells.

↓

Patient develops thirst, dyspnea on exertion, vomiting, abdominal cramps, confusion, lethargy, and hyponatremia.

Thyroid cancer

- Most common endocrine malignancy
- Occurs in all age-groups, especially in those who have had radiation treatment of the neck

Cause
- Unknown

Pathophysiologic changes

Tumor growth ➤	Painless nodule or hard nodule in an enlarged thyroid gland or palpable lymph nodes
Pressure of tumor on surrounding structures ➤	Hoarseness, dysphagia, and dyspnea
Excess thyroid hormone production ➤	Hyperthyroidism
Tumor destruction of the gland or surgical removal of the gland ➤	Hypothyroidism

EARLY, LOCALIZED THYROID CANCER

ANTERIOR VIEW

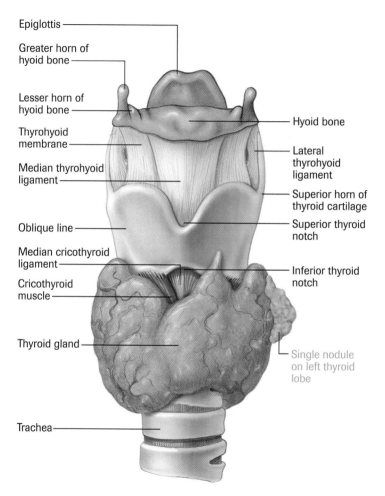

Epiglottis

Greater horn of
hyoid bone

Lesser horn of
hyoid bone

Thyrohyoid
membrane

Median thyrohyoid
ligament

Oblique line

Median cricothyroid
ligament

Cricothyroid
muscle

Thyroid gland

Trachea

Hyoid bone

Lateral
thyrohyoid
ligament

Superior horn of
thyroid cartilage

Superior thyroid
notch

Inferior thyroid
notch

Single nodule
on left thyroid
lobe

9

Renal system

Acute renal failure

- Sudden interruption of renal function
- Classified by cause: prerenal, intrarenal, or postrenal
- Three distinct phases: oliguric, diuretic, and recovery
- Usually reversible with treatment

Causes

PRERENAL
- Antihypertensive drugs; diuretic overuse
- Arrhythmias, cardiac tamponade, cardiogenic shock, heart failure, or myocardial infarction
- Arterial embolism, arterial or venous thrombosis, or hemorrhage
- Burns, sepsis, or trauma
- Dehydration; hypovolemic shock

INTRARENAL
- Crush injuries; myopathy
- Diseases of the kidney
- Nephrotoxins
- Sickle cell disease

POSTRENAL
- Bladder obstruction, urethral obstruction, or ureteral obstruction

Pathophysiologic changes

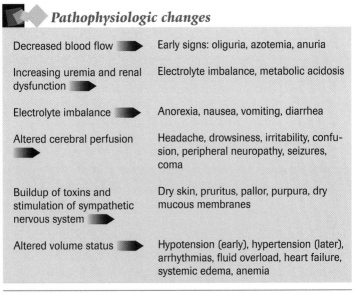

Decreased blood flow ➡	Early signs: oliguria, azotemia, anuria
Increasing uremia and renal dysfunction ➡	Electrolyte imbalance, metabolic acidosis
Electrolyte imbalance ➡	Anorexia, nausea, vomiting, diarrhea
Altered cerebral perfusion ➡	Headache, drowsiness, irritability, confusion, peripheral neuropathy, seizures, coma
Buildup of toxins and stimulation of sympathetic nervous system ➡	Dry skin, pruritus, pallor, purpura, dry mucous membranes
Altered volume status ➡	Hypotension (early), hypertension (later), arrhythmias, fluid overload, heart failure, systemic edema, anemia

MECHANISM OF ACUTE RENAL FAILURE

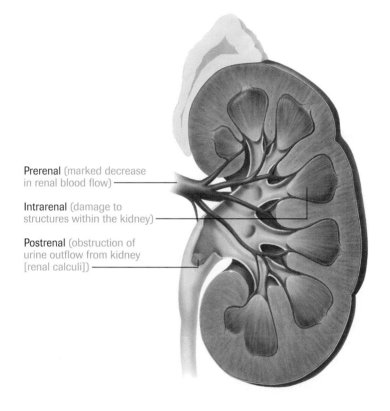

Prerenal (marked decrease in renal blood flow)

Intrarenal (damage to structures within the kidney)

Postrenal (obstruction of urine outflow from kidney [renal calculi])

Acute tubular necrosis

- Most common cause of acute renal failure
- Results from ischemia or nephrotoxicity
- Causes injury to the nephron's tubular segment, possibly leading to renal failure and uremic syndrome

Causes

ISCHEMIC INJURY

- Anesthetics, surgery, or transfusion reactions
- Cardiogenic or septic shock
- Circulatory collapse; severe hypotension
- Hemorrhage, severe dehydration, or trauma

NEPHROTOXIC INJURY

- Hypersensitivity reaction of kidneys to antibiotics or radiographic contrast agents
- Ingesting or inhaling toxic chemicals

Pathophysiologic changes

Marked decrease in glomerular filtration rate ➡	Decreased urine output, hyperkalemia, elevated serum creatinine and blood urea nitrogen (BUN) levels, dry mucous membranes and skin, central nervous system changes (lethargy, twitching, or seizures), uremic syndrome (oliguria or anuria and confusion)
Return of BUN and creatinine levels to normal (recovery phase) ➡	Diuresis

ISCHEMIC NECROSIS

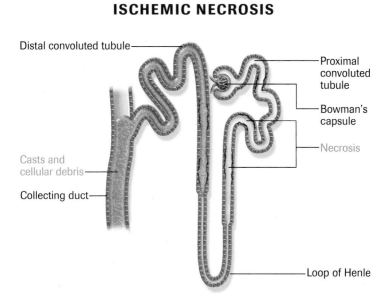

Distal convoluted tubule

Proximal convoluted tubule

Bowman's capsule

Necrosis

Casts and cellular debris

Collecting duct

Loop of Henle

NEPHROTOXIC INJURY

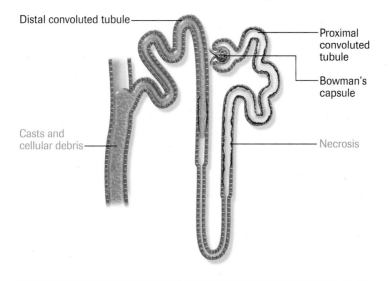

Distal convoluted tubule

Proximal convoluted tubule

Bowman's capsule

Casts and cellular debris

Necrosis

Acute tubular necrosis

Bladder cancer

- May develop on surface of bladder wall (benign or malignant papillomas) or grow within bladder wall (generally more virulent) and quickly invade underlying muscles
- Most common type: transitional cell carcinoma, arising from transitional epithelium of mucous membranes
- Less common types: adenocarcinomas, epidermoid carcinomas, squamous cell carcinomas, sarcomas, tumors in bladder diverticula, and carcinoma in situ
- Commonly asymptomatic in early stages

Cause
- Unknown

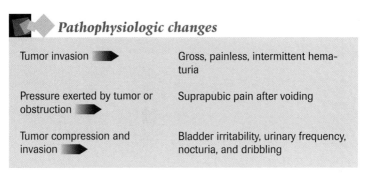

Pathophysiologic changes

Tumor invasion ➤	Gross, painless, intermittent hematuria
Pressure exerted by tumor or obstruction ➤	Suprapubic pain after voiding
Tumor compression and invasion ➤	Bladder irritability, urinary frequency, nocturia, and dribbling

BLADDER TUMOR

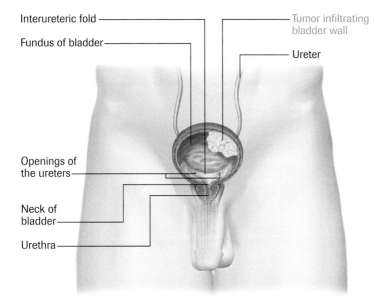

Interureteric fold

Fundus of bladder

Tumor infiltrating bladder wall

Ureter

Openings of the ureters

Neck of bladder

Urethra

Cystitis

- Lower urinary tract infection (UTI) occurring in two forms: cystitis and urethritis
- Ten times more common in women than in men
- Lower UTI also a prevalent bacterial disease in children, most commonly in girls
- Infection usually ascending from urethra to the bladder
- Usually responds readily to treatment

Causes
- Gram-negative, enteric species of bacteria (such as *Escherichia*)
- In children, commonly related to anatomical or physiologic abnormalities

Pathophysiologic changes

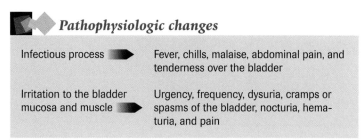

Infectious process ➤	Fever, chills, malaise, abdominal pain, and tenderness over the bladder
Irritation to the bladder mucosa and muscle ➤	Urgency, frequency, dysuria, cramps or spasms of the bladder, nocturia, hematuria, and pain

CHARACTERISTIC CHANGES IN CYSTITIS

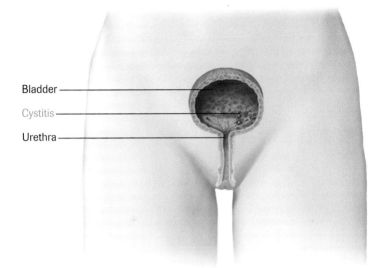

Bladder ───────
Cystitis ───────
Urethra ───────

BLADDER WALL—ENDOSCOPIC VIEW

NORMAL WALL

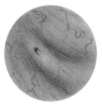

ACUTE CYSTITIS

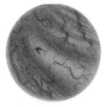

Glomerulonephritis

- Bacterial inflammation of glomeruli; may be acute or chronic
- Acute form: typically follows streptococcal infection
- Chronic form: characterized by inflammation, sclerosis, scarring and, eventually, renal failure; typically remaining undetected until progressive phase (usually irreversible)
- Rapidly progressive glomerulonephritis (RPGN): subacute, crescentic, or extracapillary glomerulonephritis; may be idiopathic or associated with proliferative glomerular disease
- Goodpasture's syndrome (rare)

Causes

ACUTE GLOMERULONEPHRITIS AND RPGN
- Immunoglobulin A nephropathy (Berger's disease)
- Impetigo
- Lipoid nephrosis
- Respiratory tract or streptococcal infection

CHRONIC GLOMERULONEPHRITIS
- Focal glomerulosclerosis
- Goodpasture's syndrome
- Hemolytic uremic syndrome
- Membranoproliferative glomerulonephritis
- Membranous glomerulopathy
- Poststreptococcal glomerulonephritis
- RPGN
- Systemic lupus erythematosus

Pathophysiologic changes

Decreased glomerular filtration rate (GFR) ➤	Decreased urination or oliguria
Hematuria ➤	Smoky or coffee colored urine
Hypervolemia ➤	Dyspnea and orthopnea, periorbital edema, bibasilar crackles
Decreased GFR, sodium or water retention, and inappropriate release of renin ➤	Mild to severe hypertension

IMMUNE COMPLEX DEPOSITS ON GLOMERULUS

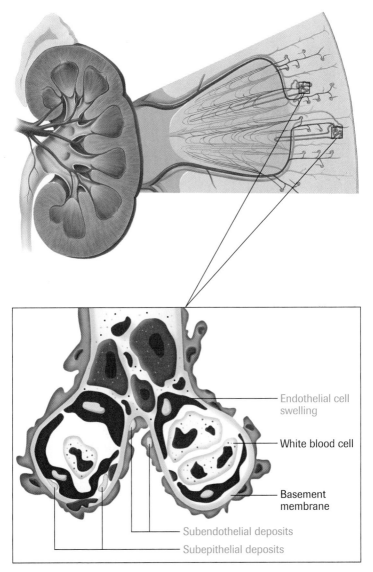

Endothelial cell swelling

White blood cell

Basement membrane

Subendothelial deposits

Subepithelial deposits

Hydronephrosis

- Abnormal dilation of the renal pelvis and the calyces of one or both kidneys, caused by an obstruction of urine flow
- Symptomatic renal dysfunction as condition progresses

Causes
- Abdominal tumors
- Benign prostatic hyperplasia
- Blood clots
- Calculi
- Congenital abnormalities
- Neurogenic bladder
- Strictures or stenosis of the ureter or bladder outlet
- Trauma
- Urethral strictures

Pathophysiologic changes

Increase in pressure above the area of obstruction in the urinary tract ➤	Severe, colicky renal pain or dull flank pain that may radiate to the groin; abdominal fullness; incomplete emptying of the bladder; dribbling; and hesitancy
Gross urinary abnormalities ➤	Hematuria, pyuria, dysuria, alternating oliguria and polyuria, or complete anuria

RENAL DAMAGE IN HYDRONEPHROSIS

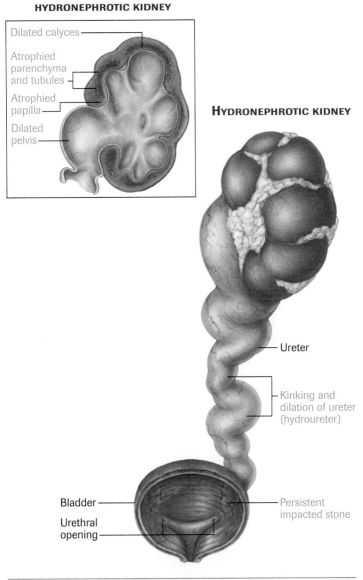

CROSS SECTION OF HYDRONEPHROTIC KIDNEY

Dilated calyces

Atrophied parenchyma and tubules

Atrophied papilla

Dilated pelvis

HYDRONEPHROTIC KIDNEY

Ureter

Kinking and dilation of ureter (hydroureter)

Bladder

Urethral opening

Persistent impacted stone

Polycystic kidney disease

- Inherited disorder characterized by multiple, bilateral, grapelike clusters of fluid-filled cysts that enlarge the kidneys, eventually replacing functioning renal tissue
- Appears in distinct infantile and adult-onset forms
- Renal deterioration more gradual in adults than infants; leads to uremia in both age-groups

Causes

- Autosomal dominant trait (adult type); three genetic variants identified
- Autosomal recessive trait (infantile type)

Pathophysiologic changes

ADULT TYPE	
Activation of the renin-angiotensin system ➤	Hypertension
Kidney enlargement ➤	Lumbar pain, widening abdominal girth, swollen and tender abdomen
INFANTILE TYPE	
Genetic abnormalities ➤	Pronounced epicanthic folds (vertical fold of skin on either side of the nose), a pointed nose, small chin, and floppy, low-set ears
Kidney enlargement ➤	Huge, bilateral, symmetrical masses on the flanks that can't be transilluminated
RENAL FAILURE	
Signs and symptoms associated with renal failure ➤	Oliguria, anuria, hyperkalemia, hypocalcemia, nausea, vomiting, peripheral edema, pruritus, anoxemia, weight gain, confusion, and fatigue

POLYCYSTIC KIDNEY

CROSS SECTION

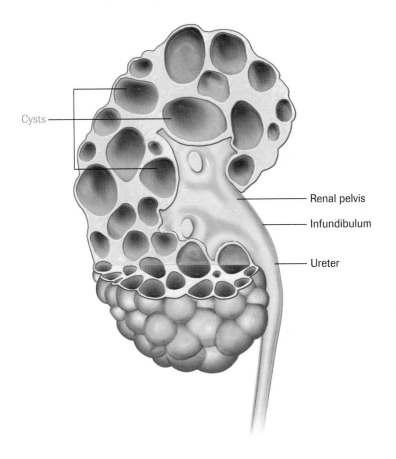

Cysts

Renal pelvis

Infundibulum

Ureter

Pyelonephritis

- Sudden inflammation caused by a bacterial infection
- Primarily affects the interstitial area and the renal pelvis or, less often, the renal tubules
- Rapid development of symptoms over a few hours to days; may resolve without treatment

Cause

- Bacterial infection (bacteria include *Escherichia coli, Proteus, Pseudomonas, Staphylococcus aureus,* or *Enterococcus faecalis*)

Pathophysiologic changes

Infectious processes ➤	Cloudy urine, fever of 102° F (38.9° C) or higher, shaking chills, flank pain, anorexia, and general malaise
Inflammation of the lower and upper urinary tract and structure ➤	Urgency, frequency, nocturia, burning during urination, dysuria, hematuria, and cloudy urine with an ammonia-like or fishy odor

PHASES OF PYELONEPHRITIS

ACUTE PYELONEPHRITIS AND PROGRESSIVE SCARRING FROM REPEATED INFECTION

3. END PHASE

Progressive scarring

Atrophied parenchyma

2. PROGRESSIVE PHASE

Focal parenchyma scarring

Narrowed calyx neck

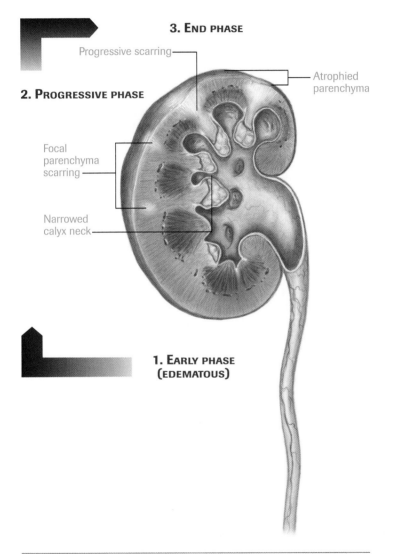

1. EARLY PHASE (EDEMATOUS)

Renal calculi

- Form anywhere in the urinary tract, although most commonly in the renal pelves or calyces
- Single or multiple stones, varying in size

Cause
- Unknown

Pathophysiologic changes

Infectious processes from urinary stasis ➡	Fever, chills, nausea, and vomiting
Obstruction by the stone ➡	Severe pain, hematuria, hydronephrosis, anuria from bilateral obstruction, and abdominal distention
Calculi traveling down a ureter ➡	Hematuria, obstruction, and severe pain

TYPES OF RENAL CALCULI

Uric acid stones

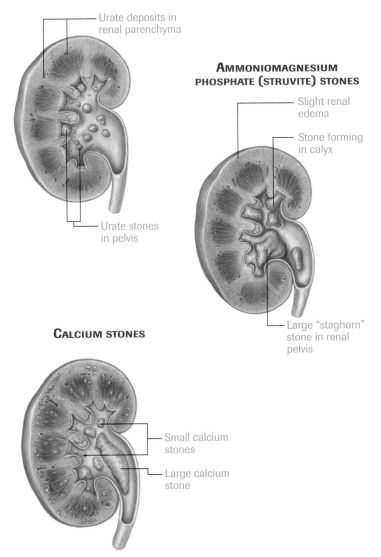

Urate deposits in
renal parenchyma

Urate stones
in pelvis

Ammoniomagnesium phosphate (struvite) stones

Slight renal
edema

Stone forming
in calyx

Large "staghorn"
stone in renal
pelvis

Calcium stones

Small calcium
stones

Large calcium
stone

Renal cancer

- Usually occurs in older adults
- Rising incidence; accounts for about 2% of all adult cancers
- Mostly occurs as metastasis from primary cancer site

Cause
- Unknown

Pathophysiologic changes

Tumor growth and pressure ➤	Constant abdominal or flank pain, palpable mass (generally smooth, firm, and nontender), obstruction of urine flow leading to urine retention
Spread of cancer to the renal pelvis ➤	Hematuria, blood clots, acute and colicky pain
Erythropoietin excess ➤	Polycythemia
Compression of renal artery with renal parenchymal ischemia and renin excess ➤	Hypertension
Renal tissue necrosis or hemorrhage ➤	Fever

TWO FORMS OF RENAL CANCER

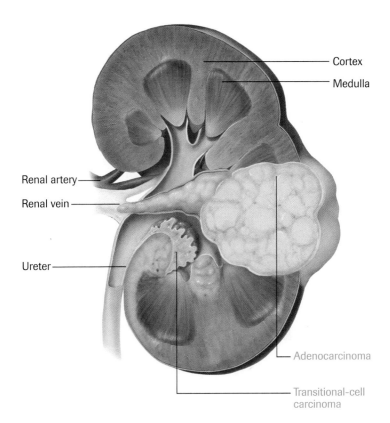

Cortex

Medulla

Renal artery

Renal vein

Ureter

Adenocarcinoma

Transitional-cell carcinoma

Renovascular hypertension

- Rise in systemic blood pressure resulting from stenosis of the major renal arteries or their branches or from intrarenal atherosclerosis
- Narrowing or sclerosis possibly partial or complete; resulting blood pressure elevation may be benign or malignant

Causes
- Anomalies of renal arteries
- Arteritis
- Atherosclerosis
- Dissecting aneurysm
- Embolism
- Fibromuscular diseases of the renal artery wall layers (fibroplasias)
- Trauma
- Tumor

Pathophysiologic changes

Release of renin ➤	Increased arterial pressures, hypertension, headache, light-headedness, retinopathy, palpitations, and tachycardia
Peripheral vasoconstriction ➤	Headache, palpitations, decreased tolerance of temperature extremes, myocardial infarction, stroke, and renal failure

RENOVASCULAR HYPERTENSION

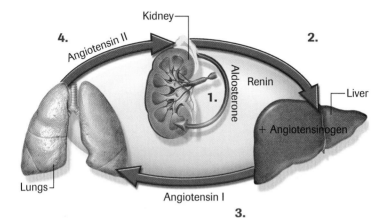

MECHANISM OF RENOVASCULAR HYPERTENSION

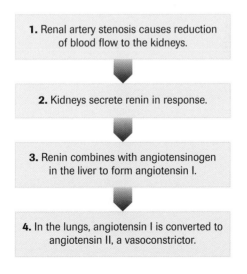

1. Renal artery stenosis causes reduction of blood flow to the kidneys.

2. Kidneys secrete renin in response.

3. Renin combines with angiotensinogen in the liver to form angiotensin I.

4. In the lungs, angiotensin I is converted to angiotensin II, a vasoconstrictor.

10

Integumentary system

Acne

- Inflammatory disease of the hair follicles associated with a high rate of sebum secretion
- Occurs on areas of the body that have sebaceous glands (face, neck, chest, back, and shoulders)
- May be inflammatory involving bacterial growth or noninflammatory

Causes
- Multifactorial-increased activity of sebaceous glands and blockage of the hair follicles

Pathophysiologic changes

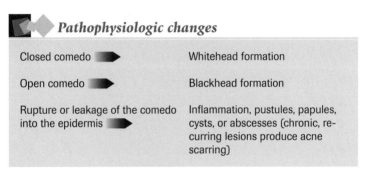

Closed comedo ➤	Whitehead formation
Open comedo ➤	Blackhead formation
Rupture or leakage of the comedo into the epidermis ➤	Inflammation, pustules, papules, cysts, or abscesses (chronic, recurring lesions produce acne scarring)

HOW ACNE DEVELOPS

EXCESSIVE SEBUM PRODUCTION

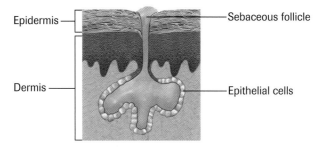

Epidermis —

Dermis —

Sebaceous follicle

Epithelial cells

INCREASED SHEDDING OF EPITHELIAL CELLS

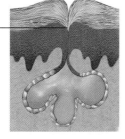

Blocked follicle—

INFLAMMATORY RESPONSE IN FOLLICLE

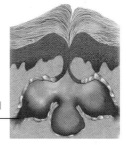

Ruptured follicle—

COMEDONES OF ACNE

CLOSED COMEDO (WHITEHEAD)

OPEN COMEDO (BLACKHEAD)

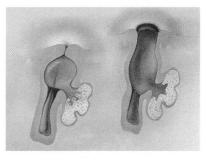

Actinic keratitis

- Premalignant lesions involving the cells of the epidermis
- Progression to squamous cell carcinoma possible if the lesions are untreated
- May disappear spontaneously or reappear after treatment

Cause
- Chronic sun damage

Pathophysiologic changes

Altered structural layer of the skin ➡	Small macule or papule with dry, rough, adherent yellow or brown scale; base may be erythematous; indurated keratoses more likely to be malignant
Distribution of macules or papules ➡	Found on sun-exposed areas: cheeks, temples, forehead, ears, neck, backs of hands, and forearms

PRECANCEROUS ACTINIC KERATOSIS

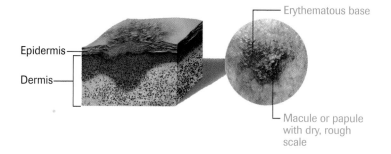

Epidermis

Dermis

Erythematous base

Macule or papule
with dry, rough
scale

Atopic dermatitis

- Chronic or recurrent inflammatory response commonly associated with bronchial asthma and allergic rhinitis
- Commonly develops in infants and toddlers between ages 1 month and 1 year and usually in those with a strong family history of atopic disease
- Generally flares and subsides and typically resolves during adolescence; may persist into adulthood

Causes
- Unknown; genetic predisposition likely
- Possible contributing factors: chemical irritants, extremes of humidity and temperature, food allergy, infection, psychological stress and strong emotions

Pathophysiologic changes

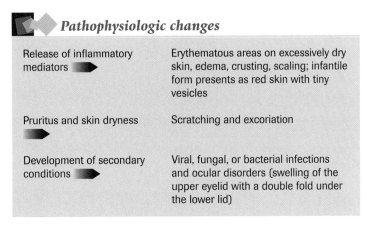

Release of inflammatory mediators ▶	Erythematous areas on excessively dry skin, edema, crusting, scaling; infantile form presents as red skin with tiny vesicles
Pruritus and skin dryness ▶	Scratching and excoriation
Development of secondary conditions ▶	Viral, fungal, or bacterial infections and ocular disorders (swelling of the upper eyelid with a double fold under the lower lid)

APPEARANCE OF ATOPIC DERMATITIS

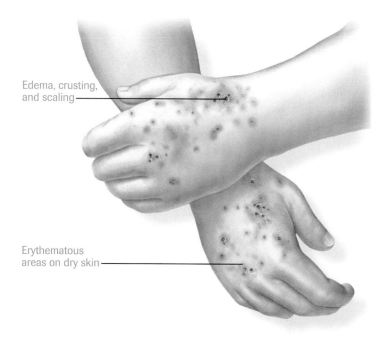

Edema, crusting, and scaling

Erythematous areas on dry skin

Basal cell carcinoma

- Slow-growing, destructive skin tumor; also called *basal cell epithelioma*
- Accounts for more than 50% of all cancers
- Changes in the epidermal basal cells diminishing maturation and normal keratinization; continuing division of basal cells leads to mass formation

Causes
- Prolonged sun exposure (most common)
- Arsenic, burns, immunosuppression, radiation exposure, and vaccinations (rare)

Pathophysiologic changes

NODULO-ULCERATIVE LESIONS

Unrepaired mutations in skin cells ➡

Appearing most commonly on the face

Early stages: small lesions; smooth, pinkish, translucent papules; telangiectatic vessels cross surface; lesions occasionally pigmented

As lesions enlarge, depressed center with firm, elevated borders

Ulceration and local invasion, possibly causing massive hemorrhage (if invasion of large blood vessels)

SUPERFICIAL BASAL CELL CARCINOMA

Unrepaired mutations in skin cells ➡

Typically numerous and commonly occurring on the chest and back

Oval or irregular shaped, lightly pigmented plaques, with sharply defined, slightly elevated, threadlike borders

Superficial erosion

SCLEROSING BASAL CELL CARCINOMA

Unrepaired mutations in skin cells ➡

Occurring on head and neck

Lesions appearing waxy, sclerotic, yellow to white plaques, without distinct borders

BASAL CELL CARCINOMA

Central crater ——————— ——————— Papule

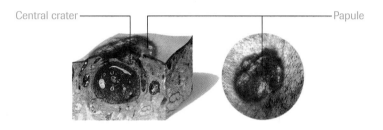

Burns

- Classified as first degree, second-degree superficial, second-degree deep partial thickness, third-degree full thickness, and fourth degree
- Survival rate dependent on immediate, aggressive burn treatment

Causes
- Abrasion or friction
- Chemical: contact, ingestion, inhalation, or injection of acids, alkalis, or vesicants
- Electrical: contact with faulty electrical cords, electrical wiring, or high-voltage power lines
- Thermal: automobile accidents, residential fires, or scalds caused by bathroom or kitchen accidents or child abuse
- Ultraviolet radiation: sunburn

Pathophysiologic changes

FIRST-DEGREE BURN

Epidermal destruction ➡	Localized pain and erythema, usually without blisters in the first 24 hours
Fluid shift ➡	Chills, headache, localized edema, and nausea and vomiting

SECOND-DEGREE BURN

Epidermal and some dermal destruction ➡	Thin-walled, fluid-filled blisters appearing within minutes of injury; mild to moderate edema and pain
Epidermal and full dermal destruction ➡	White, waxy appearance to damaged area

THIRD- AND FOURTH-DEGREE BURN

Epidermal, dermal, subcutaneous tissue, and muscle destruction ➡	White, brown, or black leathery tissue and visible thrombosed vessels
Fluid shifts ➡	Edema, hemodynamic instability
Catecholamine secretion ➡	Increased metabolic rate, protein and fat wasting
Loss of intact skin ➡	Infection and spesis

CLASSIFICATION OF BURNS BY DEPTH OF INJURY

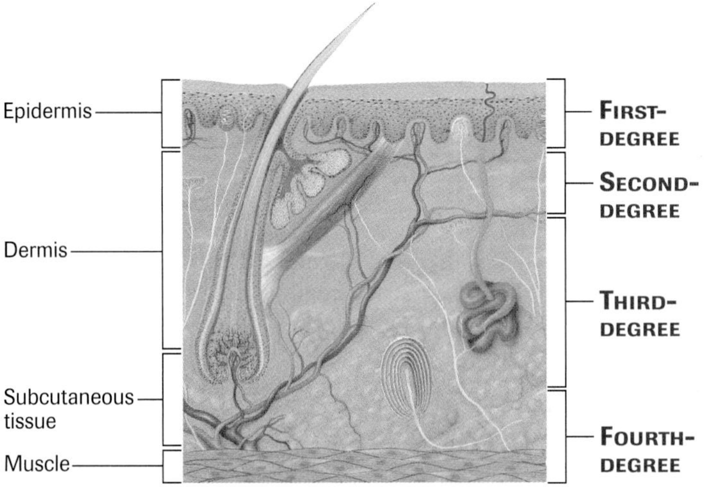

Epidermis

Dermis

Subcutaneous tissue

Muscle

FIRST-DEGREE

SECOND-DEGREE

THIRD-DEGREE

FOURTH-DEGREE

Cellulitis

- Infection of dermis or subcutaneous layer of skin, possibly resulting from skin damage (bite or wound)
- May cause fever, erythema, or lymphangitis
- Risk factors: diabetes, immunodeficiency, impaired circulation, neuropathy

Causes

- Bacterial and fungal infections, commonly group A beta-hemolytic streptococcus or *Staphylococcus aureus*
- In diabetes or decreased immune function: *Acinetobacter, Cryptococcus neoformans, Enterobacter, Escherichia coli, Mycobacterium fortuitum* complex, *Pasteurella multocida, Proteus mirabilis, Pseudomonas aeruginosa,* and *Vibrio vulnificus*
- In children, less commonly caused by pneumococci and *Neisseria meningitidis* group B (periorbital)

Pathophysiologic changes

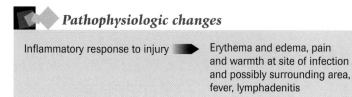

Inflammatory response to injury ➡ Erythema and edema, pain and warmth at site of infection and possibly surrounding area, fever, lymphadenitis

PHASES OF ACUTE INFLAMMATORY RESPONSE

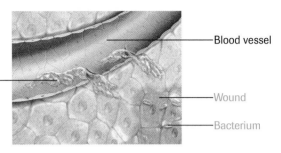

Increased blood flow carrying plasma proteins and fluid to the injured tissue

Blood vessel

Wound

Bacterium

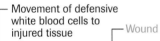

Movement of defensive white blood cells to injured tissue

Wound

Wound

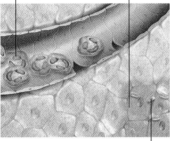

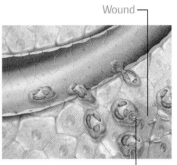

Bacterium

Phagocyte engulfing bacterium

RECOGNIZING CELLULITIS

The classic signs of cellulitis are erythema and edema surrounding the initial wound. The tissue is warm to the touch.

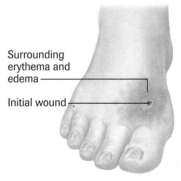

Surrounding erythema and edema

Initial wound

Contact dermatitis

- Sharply demarcated inflammation of skin
- Results from contact with irritating chemical or atopic allergen
- Produces varying symptoms, depending on type and degree of exposure

Causes
- Allergens: sensitization after repeated exposure
- Mild irritants: chronic exposure to detergents or solvents
- Strong irritants: damage or contact with acids or alkalis

Pathophysiologic changes

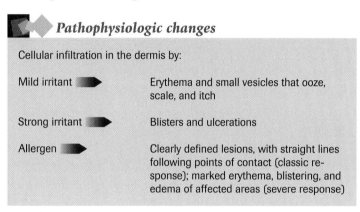

Cellular infiltration in the dermis by:

Mild irritant ➤	Erythema and small vesicles that ooze, scale, and itch
Strong irritant ➤	Blisters and ulcerations
Allergen ➤	Clearly defined lesions, with straight lines following points of contact (classic response); marked erythema, blistering, and edema of affected areas (severe response)

WHAT HAPPENS IN CONTACT DERMATITIS

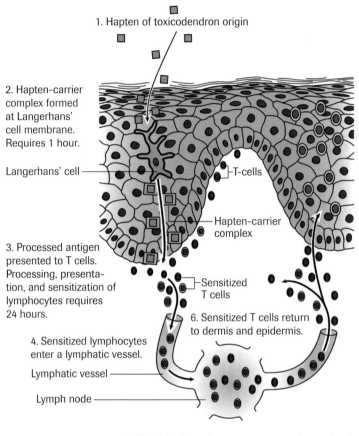

1. Hapten of toxicodendron origin

2. Hapten-carrier complex formed at Langerhans' cell membrane. Requires 1 hour.

Langerhans' cell

T-cells

Hapten-carrier complex

3. Processed antigen presented to T cells. Processing, presentation, and sensitization of lymphocytes requires 24 hours.

Sensitized T cells

6. Sensitized T cells return to dermis and epidermis.

4. Sensitized lymphocytes enter a lymphatic vessel.

Lymphatic vessel

Lymph node

5. Sensitized lymphocytes transported to regional lymph nodes, where T cell hyperplasia is induced.

Image from Ruben, E.M.D., and Farber J.L., MD. *Pathology,* 3rd ed. Philadelphia: Lippincott Williams & Wilkins, 1999.

Herpes zoster

- Acute inflammation caused by infection with herpesvirus varicella-zoster (chickenpox virus); also called *shingles*
- Produces localized vesicular skin lesions and severe neuralgic pain in peripheral areas
- Usually occurs in adults
- Complete recovery common, but may cause scarring, vision impairment (with corneal damage), or persistent neuralgia

Cause

- Reactivation of varicella-zoster virus

Pathophysiologic changes

Viral reactivation ➤	Fever and malaise; eruption of small, red, nodular skin lesions on painful areas
Innervation of nerves arising in inflamed root ganglia ➤	Severe, deep pain; pruritus; paresthesia or hyperesthesia
	Usually developing on trunk; occasionally on arms and legs in dermatomal distribution
	Pain may be continuous or intermittent; usually lasting 1 to 4 weeks
Trigeminal ganglion involvement ➤	Eye pain, corneal and scleral damage, and impaired vision
Oculomotor involvement (rare) ➤	Conjunctivitis, extraocular weakness, ptosis, and paralytic mydriasis

HERPES ZOSTER

Erythematous base

Umbilicated vesicles

From Goodheart, H.P., MD. *Goodheart's Photoguide of Common Skin Disorders,* 2nd ed. Philadelphia: Lippincott Williams & Wilkins, 2003.

Malignant melanoma

- Neoplasm arising from melanocytes; characterized by enlargement of skin lesion or nevus accompanied by changes in color, inflammation, soreness, itching, ulceration, bleeding, or texture
- Common sites: head and neck (men), legs (women), and back
- Classified as superficial spreading melanoma, nodular malignant melanoma, lentigo maligna melanoma, and acral-lentiginous melanoma

Cause

- Excessive exposure to sunlight

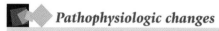 *Pathophysiologic changes*

SUPERFICIAL SPREADING MELANOMA

Mutation in melanin-producing cells of skin ➡ Appearing as red, white, or blue in color over brown or black background, with irregular notched margin

Appearing as irregular, small, elevated tumor nodules that may ulcerate and bleed

NODULAR MALIGNANT MELANOMA

Mutation in melanin-producing cells of skin ➡ Resembling blood blister or polyp and possibly appearing anywhere on the body

LENTIGO MALIGNA MELANOMA

Mutation in melanin-producing cells of skin ➡ Resembling large, flat freckle typically brown, black, whitish, or slate color, with irregularly scattered black nodules on the surface

ACRAL-LENTIGINOUS MELANOMA

Mutation in melanin-producing cells of skin ➡ Developing as irregular, enlarging black macule; occurring mainly on the palms and soles

MALIGNANT MELANOMA

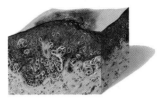

- Can arise on normal skin or from an existing mole
- If not treated promptly, can spread to other areas of skin, lymph nodes, or internal organs

ABCDEs OF MALIGNANT MELANOMA

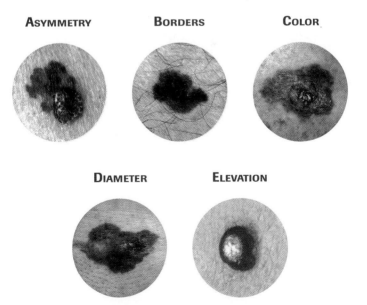

ASYMMETRY

BORDERS

COLOR

DIAMETER

ELEVATION

Pressure ulcers

- Localized areas of cellular necrosis occurring in the skin and subcutaneous tissue over bony prominences
- Characterized as superficial or deep
- Categorized as stage I, stage II, stage III, or stage IV

Causes

- Constant moisture on the skin, causing tissue maceration
- Friction and shear, causing damage to the epidermal and upper dermal skin layers
- Immobility and decreased level of activity
- Impaired hygiene, as with fecal incontinence, leading to skin breakdown

Pathophysiologic changes

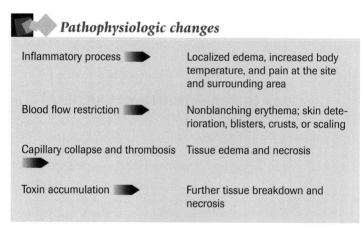

Inflammatory process ➤	Localized edema, increased body temperature, and pain at the site and surrounding area
Blood flow restriction ➤	Nonblanching erythema; skin deterioration, blisters, crusts, or scaling
Capillary collapse and thrombosis ➤	Tissue edema and necrosis
Toxin accumulation ➤	Further tissue breakdown and necrosis

PRESSURE ULCER STAGES

Stage I

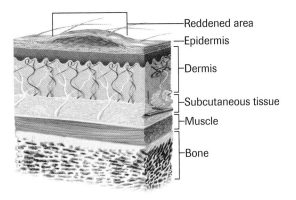

- Reddened area
- Epidermis
- Dermis
- Subcutaneous tissue
- Muscle
- Bone

Stage II	Stage III	Stage IV

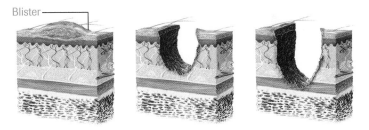

Blister

Psoriasis

- Chronic, recurrent disease characterized by epidermal proliferation, with recurring partial remissions and exacerbations
- Flare-ups commonly related to specific systemic and environmental factors but may be unpredictable
- Widespread involvement indicated by exfoliative and erythrodermic psoriasis

Causes

- Flare-up of drop-shaped lesions from infections, especially beta-hemolytic streptococci
- Genetic factors
- Possible immune disorder

Pathophysiologic changes

Immune-based inflammatory reaction by T cells in dermis ➤	Erythematous and usually well-defined plaques, sometimes covering large areas of the body (psoriatic lesions)
	Lesions most commonly appearing on scalp, chest, elbows, knees, back, and buttocks
	Plaques have characteristic silver scales that either flake off easily or thicken, covering the lesion
Dry, encrusted lesions ➤	Itching and occasional pain

PSORIATIC LESION

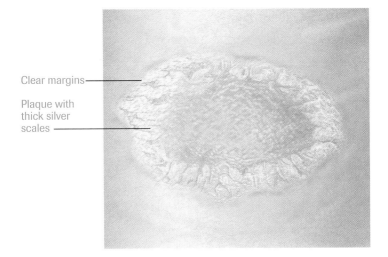

Clear margins

Plaque with
thick silver
scales

DIFFUSE PSORIATIC PLAQUES

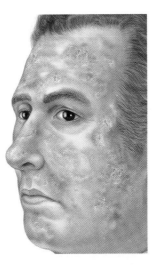

Seborrheic keratosis

■ Benign skin condition presenting as wartlike growths typically brown or black in color, although some appearing waxy or yellow
■ Lesions commonly on the back or face
■ Nonmalignant condition; not precancerous
■ May be single or appear as clusters
■ Has a pasted-on appearance

Cause
■ Unknown; suspected hereditary link

Pathophysiologic changes

Inflammation of affected areas	Itchiness, redness, and lesions rubbing or snagging clothing
Varying degrees of pigmentation	Lesions appearing tan, brown, black, yellow, or waxy

SEBORRHEIC KERATOSIS

BASAL CELL PAPILLOMA

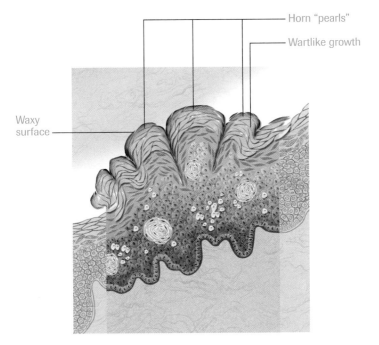

Horn "pearls"

Wartlike growth

Waxy surface

Squamous cell carcinoma

- Invasive tumor with metastatic potential arising from keratinizing epidermal cells
- Occurs most commonly in fair-skinned white men older than age 60
- Higher incidence with outdoor employment or residence in sunny, warm climate

Causes

- Chronic skin inflammation and irritation
- Hereditary diseases
- Ingested herbicides, medications, or waxes containing arsenic
- Local carcinogens, such as oil and tar
- Overexposure to the sun's ultraviolet rays
- Premalignant lesions, such as actinic keratosis or leukoplakia
- X-ray therapy

Pathophysiologic changes

Mutation in keratinizing epidermal cells of skin ➤	Nodule with firm, indurated base
Inflammation and induration of lesion ➤	Early lesions: scaling and ulceration of opaque, firm nodules with indistinct borders; possibly appearing on face, ear, dorsa of hand and forearm, or other sun-damaged area
Keratinization ➤	Later lesions: scaly; most commonly appearing on face and hands; lesions on lower lip or ear possibly indicating invasive metastasis
Metastasis to regional lymph nodes ➤	Pain, malaise, fatigue, weakness, and anorexia

SQUAMOUS CELL CARCINOMA

Early firm,
red nodule

Untreated
nodule
spreading

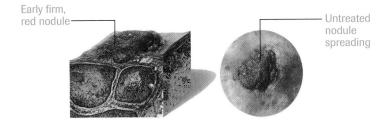

Urticaria

- Episodic skin reaction characterized by local dermal wheals surrounded by an erythematous flare (also known as *hives*)
- May be intermittent and self-limited or chronic
- Symptoms lasting less than 6 weeks characterized as acute; symptoms lasting longer than 6 weeks characterized as chronic

Causes

- Allergic: aeroallergens and drugs, food, insect bites and stings
- Nonallergic: external physical stimuli, hereditary influences, and infection

Pathophysiologic changes

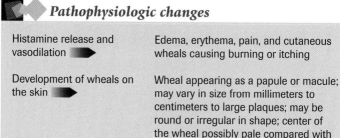

Histamine release and vasodilation ➡	Edema, erythema, pain, and cutaneous wheals causing burning or itching
Development of wheals on the skin ➡	Wheal appearing as a papule or macule; may vary in size from millimeters to centimeters to large plaques; may be round or irregular in shape; center of the wheal possibly pale compared with the erythematous tissue surrounding the wheal; a halo effect possibly present around the wheal

URTICARIA (HIVES)

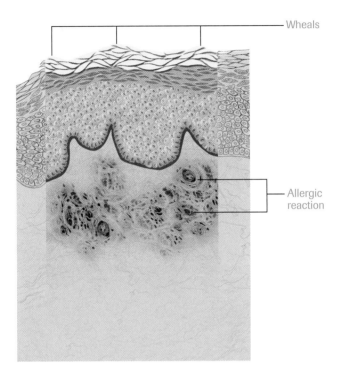

Wheals

Allergic
reaction

Warts

- Common, benign, viral infections of the skin and adjacent mucous membranes
- May disappear spontaneously, or with treatment, or require vigorous and prolonged treatment

Causes
- Human papillomavirus
- Probably transmitted through direct contact; autoinoculation

Pathophysiologic changes

Replication of the epidermal cells ➡	Lesions with varying characteristics; may be rough or smooth, rounded or irregularly shaped, elevated or flat, single or multiple groupings, dry or moist, soft or coarse, and possibly occurring on any part of the body

CROSS SECTION OF A WART

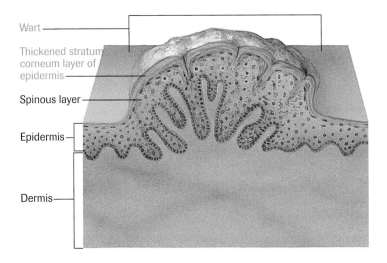

Wart

Thickened stratum corneum layer of epidermis

Spinous layer

Epidermis

Dermis

PERIUNGUAL WARTS

Warts around the edges of fingernails and toenails are rough and irregularly shaped, and they have an elevated surface. A severe wart may extend under the nail and lift it off the nail bed, causing pain.

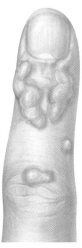

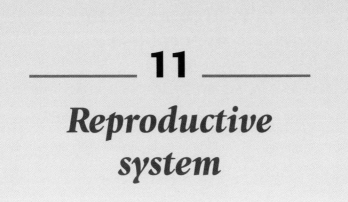

11

Reproductive system

Benign prostatic hyperplasia

- Characterized by an enlarged prostate gland and a compressed urethra, causing overt urinary obstruction; also known as *benign prostatic hypertrophy*
- Typically associated with aging (most men over age 50 having some prostatic enlargement)
- Treated symptomatically or surgically, depending on the prostate's size, the patient's age and health, and the extent of the obstruction

Causes
- Exact cause unknown
- Possible age-related changes in hormone activity; androgenic hormone production decreasing with age, causing an imbalance in androgen and estrogen levels and a high level of dihydrotestosterone (main prostatic intracellular androgen)

Pathophysiologic changes

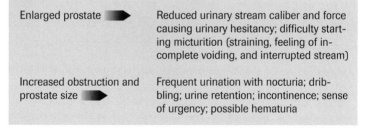

Enlarged prostate ➡	Reduced urinary stream caliber and force causing urinary hesitancy; difficulty starting micturition (straining, feeling of incomplete voiding, and interrupted stream)
Increased obstruction and prostate size ➡	Frequent urination with nocturia; dribbling; urine retention; incontinence; sense of urgency; possible hematuria

PROSTATIC ENLARGEMENT

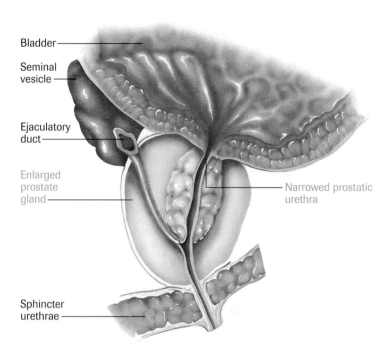

Bladder

Seminal
vesicle

Ejaculatory
duct

Enlarged
prostate
gland

Narrowed prostatic
urethra

Sphincter
urethrae

Breast cancer

- Most common cancer affecting women
- May develop any time after puberty, usually after age 50

Causes
- Unknown

Pathophysiologic changes

Mutation in breast tissue cells ➤	Lump or mass in breast (hard, stony mass usually malignant); change in breast size or symmetry; change in nipple (itching, burning, erosion, or retraction); and nipple discharge (watery, serous, creamy, bloody)
Fixation of cancer to pectoral muscles or underlying fascia ➤	Change in breast skin (thickening, scaly skin around nipple, dimpling)
Edema ➤	Change in skin texture (peau d'orange)
Advancing spread within breast ➤	Change in skin temperature (warm, hot, or pink area), ulceration, edema, or pain (not usually present; should be investigated)
Metastasis ➤	Pathologic bone fractures; edema of arm

UNDERSTANDING BREAST CANCER

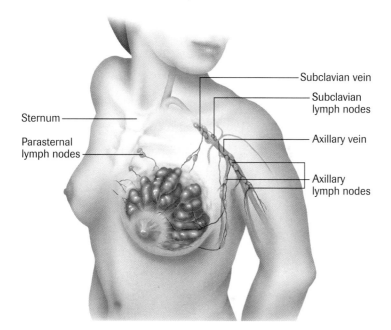

Subclavian vein

Subclavian lymph nodes

Sternum

Parasternal lymph nodes

Axillary vein

Axillary lymph nodes

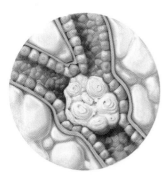

DUCTAL CARCINOMA IN SITU

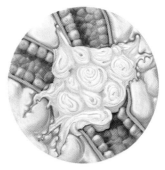

INFILTRATING (INVASIVE) DUCTAL CARCINOMA

Cervical cancer

- Third most common cancer of the female reproductive system
- Classified as either microinvasive or invasive
- Precancerous dysplasia: occurs more frequently than invasive cancer and more often in younger women
- Invasive carcinoma: occurs in women ages 30 to 50; rare in those under age 20

Causes
- Unknown

Pathophysiologic changes

Cellular invasion and erosion of the cervical epithelium ➤	Abnormal vaginal bleeding with persistent vaginal discharge and postcoital pain and bleeding
Pressure on the surrounding tissues and nerves from cellular proliferation ➤	Pelvic pain
Erosion and necrosis of the cervix ➤	Vaginal leakage of urine and feces from fistulas
Cellular proliferation and increased tumor growth needs ➤	Anorexia, weight loss, and anemia

CERVICAL CANCER

CARCINOMA IN SITU

SQUAMOUS CELL CARCINOMA

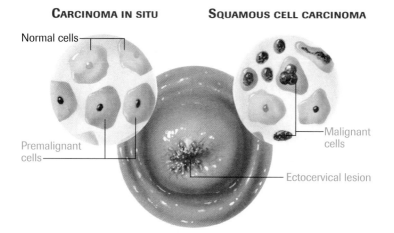

Normal cells

Premalignant cells

Malignant cells

Ectocervical lesion

PAP SMEAR FINDINGS

NORMAL
- Large, surface-type squamous cells
- Small, pyknotic nuclei

MILD DYSPLASIA
- Mild increase in nuclear : cytoplasmic ratio
- Hyperchromatism
- Abnormal chromatin pattern

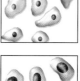

SEVERE DYSPLASIA, CARCINOMA IN SITU
- Basal type cells
- Very high nuclear : cytoplasmic ratio
- Marked hyperchromatism
- Abnormal chromatin

INVASIVE CARCINOMA
- Marked pleomorphism
- Irregular nuclei
- Clumped chromatin
- Prominent nucleoli

Endometrial cancer

- Also known as *uterine cancer*
- Most common gynecological cancer
- Usually affects postmenopausal women ages 50 to 60
- In most premenopausal women who develop uterine cancer: history of anovulatory menstrual cycles or other hormone imbalance

Causes
- Unknown

Pathophysiologic changes

Tumor growth ➤	Uterine enlargement, pain
Erosive effects of tumor growth ➤	Persistent and unusual premenopausal bleeding or postmenopausal bleeding
Progressive infiltration and invasion of tumor cells and continued cellular proliferation ➤	Pain, weight loss

PROGRESSION OF ENDOMETRIAL CANCER

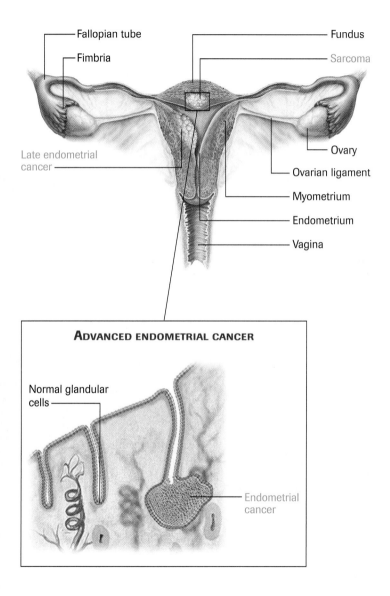

Fallopian tube

Fimbria

Fundus

Sarcoma

Late endometrial cancer

Ovary

Ovarian ligament

Myometrium

Endometrium

Vagina

ADVANCED ENDOMETRIAL CANCER

Normal glandular cells

Endometrial cancer

Endometriosis

- Presence of endometrial tissue outside the lining of the uterine cavity
- Generally confined to pelvic area (usually around the ovaries, uterovesical peritoneum, uterosacral ligaments, and cul de sac) but may appear anywhere in the body (including intestines, even found in lungs and limbs)

Causes
- Unknown

Pathophysiologic changes

Implantation of ectopic tissue and adhesions ➤	Dysmenorrhea (pain typically beginning 5 to 7 days before menses, lasting for 2 to 3 days after peak of menses)
Ectopic tissue in ovaries and oviducts ➤	Infertility and profuse menses
Ectopic tissue in ovaries or cul de sac ➤	Deep-thrust dyspareunia
Ectopic tissue in bladder ➤	Suprapubic pain, dysuria, and hematuria
Ectopic tissue in large bowel and appendix ➤	Abdominal cramps, pain on defecation, constipation; bloody stools (from bleeding of ectopic endometrium in rectosigmoid musculature)
Ectopic tissue in cervix, vagina, and peritoneum ➤	Bleeding from endometrial deposits during menses; painful intercourse

PELVIC ENDOMETRIOSIS

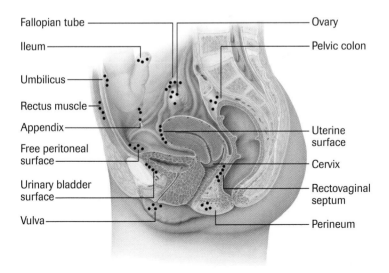

Uterus

Endometriosis over ureter

Endometrial implants

Ovary

Ruptured endometrial cyst of right ovary

COMMON SITES OF ENDOMETRIOSIS

Fallopian tube

Ileum

Umbilicus

Rectus muscle

Appendix

Free peritoneal surface

Urinary bladder surface

Vulva

Ovary

Pelvic colon

Uterine surface

Cervix

Rectovaginal septum

Perineum

Fibroid disease
of the uterus

- Uterine leiomyomas most common benign tumors in women
- Most common in the uterine corpus, although may appear on the cervix or on the round or broad ligament
- May be present in 15% to 20% of reproductive women and 30% to 40% of women over age 30

Causes
- Unknown

Pathophysiologic changes

Disrupted endometrial cavity vessels due to uterine cavity growth ➤	Abnormal bleeding (most common symptom)
Tumor growth ➤	Pain, pelvic pressure, impingement on adjacent viscera, mild hyponephrosis
Fibroid outgrows the available blood supply ➤	Pain, tumor shrinkage

UTERINE FIBROIDS

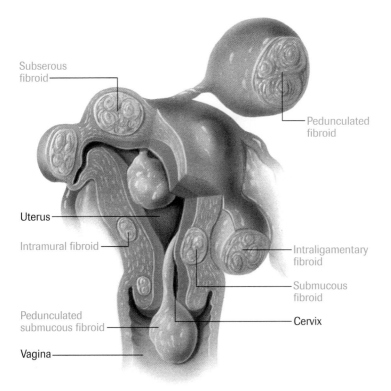

Subserous fibroid

Pedunculated fibroid

Uterus

Intramural fibroid

Intraligamentary fibroid

Submucous fibroid

Pedunculated submucous fibroid

Cervix

Vagina

Herpes simplex type 2

- Recurrent viral infection caused by *Herpesvirus hominis*
- Also known as *genital herpes;* primarily affects the genital area; commonly transmitted by sexual contact; cross-infection possible from orogenital sex
- Characterized by painful, fluid-filled vesicles appearing in genital area (some cases remaining subclinical, with no symptoms)
- Treatment largely supportive; no known cure

Causes

- Pregnancy-related transmission (Infected pregnant patient may transmit virus to neonate during vaginal delivery; cesarean section recommended during initial infection when active lesions are present.)
- Transmission of *H. hominis* (causes type 1 and type 2 herpes)
  - Primarily by sexual contact
  - Possibly by autoinoculation with type 1 herpes (through poor hand-washing practices or orogenital sex)

Pathophysiologic changes

Viral penetration of skin, viral replication, and entry into cutaneous neurons ➤	Initial symptoms: pain, tingling and itching in genital area, followed by eruption of localized fluid-filled vesicles
Painful lesions ➤	Dysuria and dyspareunia
Progression of viral infection ➤	Malaise, fever, leukorrhea (in females), and lymphadenopathy

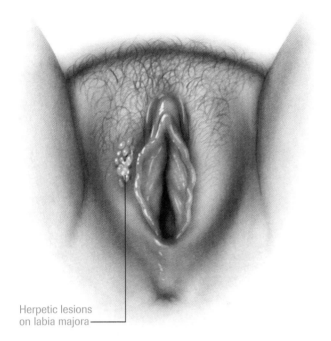

Herpetic lesions
on labia majora

Hydrocele

- Collection of fluid between the visceral and parietal layers of the tunica vaginalis of the testicle or along the spermatic cord
- Most common cause of scrotal swelling
- Congenital form: commonly resolves spontaneously during the first year of life with no treatment

Causes

- Congenital malformation (infants)
- Infection of the testes or epididymis
- Testicular tumor
- Trauma to the testes or epididymis

Pathophysiologic changes

Peritoneal fluid collection in the scrotum ➤	Scrotal swelling, feeling of heaviness, flaccid or tense mass, scrotal tenderness
Acute epididymal infection or testicular torsion ➤	Pain, swelling

HYDROCELE

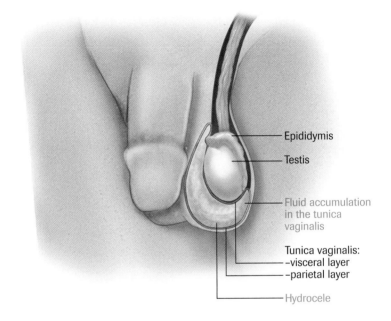

Epididymis

Testis

Fluid accumulation in the tunica vaginalis

Tunica vaginalis:
–visceral layer
–parietal layer

Hydrocele

Intraductal papilloma

- Small, benign tumor growing within a milk duct of the breast
- Occurs most commonly in women ages 35 to 55
- Usually causes discharge from a single breast duct
- Mass usually too small to be palpated

Causes
- Unknown

Pathophysiologic changes

Development of a small mass in the breast duct and epithelial overgrowth ➡	Single or multiple mass, appearing as well-defined, nonpalpable and non-mobile, firm or soft, usually nontender
Increasing pressure in the breast duct ➡	Serous, bloody nipple discharge

INTRADUCTAL PAPILLOMA

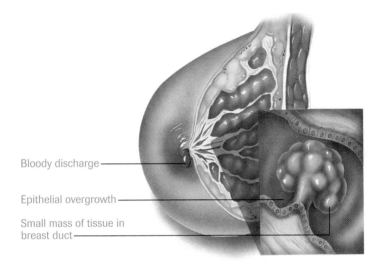

Bloody discharge

Epithelial overgrowth

Small mass of tissue in
breast duct

Ovarian cancer

- Fifth leading cause of death among U.S. women: carries the highest mortality of all gynecologic cancers
- Prognosis dependent on histologic type and stage of the disease, but generally poor because ovarian tumors produce few signs; usually advanced at diagnosis
- In women with previously treated breast cancer: metastatic ovarian cancer more common than cancer at any other site

Causes
- Unknown

Pathophysiologic changes

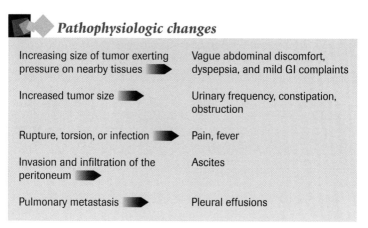

Increasing size of tumor exerting pressure on nearby tissues ➤	Vague abdominal discomfort, dyspepsia, and mild GI complaints
Increased tumor size ➤	Urinary frequency, constipation, obstruction
Rupture, torsion, or infection ➤	Pain, fever
Invasion and infiltration of the peritoneum ➤	Ascites
Pulmonary metastasis ➤	Pleural effusions

OVARIAN CANCER

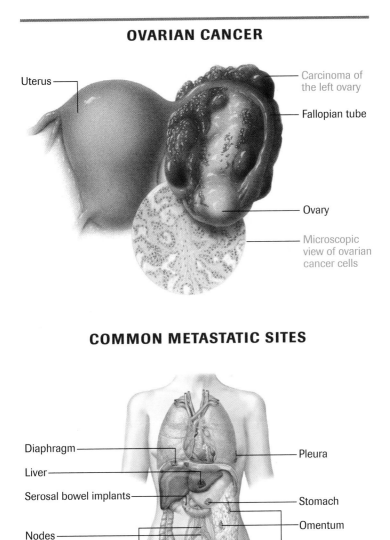

Uterus

Carcinoma of the left ovary

Fallopian tube

Ovary

Microscopic view of ovarian cancer cells

COMMON METASTATIC SITES

Diaphragm

Liver

Serosal bowel implants

Nodes

Colon

Ovaries

Pleura

Stomach

Omentum

Pelvic peritoneal implant

Ovarian cysts

- Benign sacs containing fluid or semisolid material
- Usually small and producing no symptoms, but requiring investigation as possible sites of malignant change
- May be single or multiple and generally arise during the ovulatory process
- Excellent prognosis

Causes

- Granulosa-lutein cysts (occurring within the corpus luteum): excessive accumulation of blood during hemorrhagic phase of menstrual cycle
- Theca-lutein cysts:
  - Hydatidiform mole, choriocarcinoma
  - Hormone therapy (human chorionic gonadotropin or clomiphene citrate)

Pathophysiologic changes

Large or multiple cysts ➤	Mild pelvic pain, discomfort, low back pain, dyspareunia, abnormal uterine bleeding
Cyst with torsion ➤	Acute abdominal pain
Granulosa-lutein cysts ➤	In pregnancy: unilateral pelvic discomfort
	In nonpregnant women: delayed menses, followed by prolonged or irregular bleeding

OVARIAN CYSTS

FOLLICULAR CYST

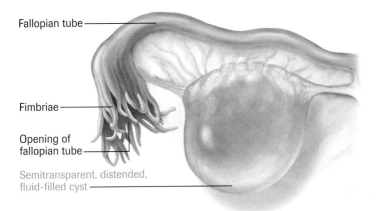

Fallopian tube

Fimbriae

Opening of fallopian tube

Semitransparent, distended, fluid-filled cyst

DERMOID CYST

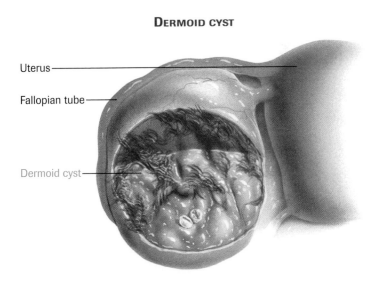

Uterus

Fallopian tube

Dermoid cyst

Pelvic inflammatory disease

- Infection in the uterus, fallopian tubes, or ovaries
- Good prognosis with early diagnosis and treatment
- Untreated, may cause infertility and potentially fatal septicemia and shock
- Chronic complications possible, including chronic pelvic pain and formation of scar tissue

Causes

- Infection with aerobic and anaerobic organisms, such as:
  - *Neisseria gonorrhoeae* and *Chlamydia trachomatis* (most common)
  - Staphylococci, streptococci, diphtheroids, *Pseudomonas, Escherichia coli*

Pathophysiologic changes

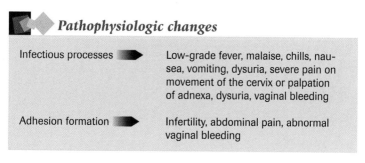

Infectious processes ➡ Low-grade fever, malaise, chills, nausea, vomiting, dysuria, severe pain on movement of the cervix or palpation of adnexa, dysuria, vaginal bleeding

Adhesion formation ➡ Infertility, abdominal pain, abnormal vaginal bleeding

DISTRIBUTION OF ADHESIONS IN PELVIC INFLAMMATORY DISEASE

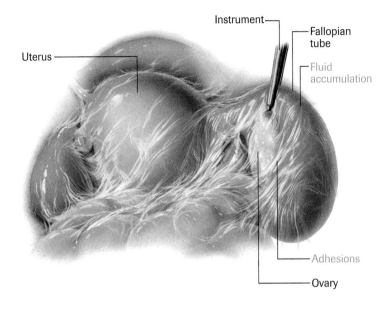

Uterus

Instrument

Fallopian tube

Fluid accumulation

Adhesions

Ovary

Prostate cancer

- Slow-growing, most common neoplasm in men over age 50
- Commonly forms as adenocarcinoma (derived from glandular tissue); sarcomas rare
- Usually originates in posterior prostate gland; sometimes originating near urethra
- Seldom results from benign hyperplastic enlargement common with aging
- Clinical manifestation typically associated with later stages of disease

Causes
- Unknown

Pathophysiologic changes

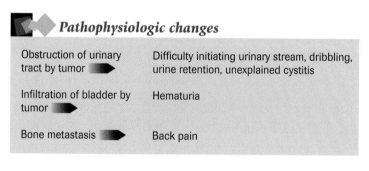

Obstruction of urinary tract by tumor ➡	Difficulty initiating urinary stream, dribbling, urine retention, unexplained cystitis
Infiltration of bladder by tumor ➡	Hematuria
Bone metastasis ➡	Back pain

PROSTATE CANCER

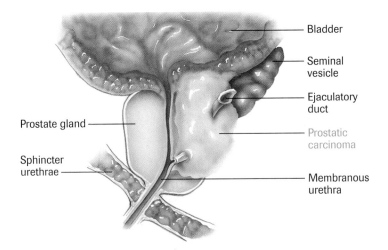

Bladder

Seminal vesicle

Ejaculatory duct

Prostate gland

Prostatic carcinoma

Sphincter urethrae

Membranous urethra

PATHWAY FOR METASTASIS OF PROSTATE CANCER

When primary prostatic lesions metastasize, they typically invade the prostatic capsule, spreading along the ejaculatory ducts in the space between the seminal vesicles or perivesicular fascia.

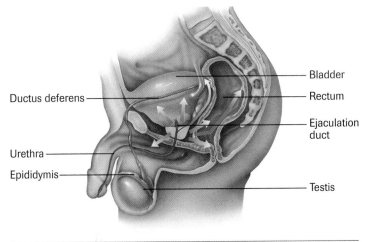

Ductus deferens

Bladder

Rectum

Ejaculation duct

Urethra

Epididymis

Testis

Prostatitis

- Inflammation of the prostate gland; may be acute or chronic
- Usually nonbacterial and idiopathic in origin
- Acute prostatitis: easily recognized and treated
- Chronic prostatitis: most common cause of recurrent urinary tract infections (UTIs) in men; less easily recognized

Causes

- Bacterial prostatitis — *Escherichia coli*, *Klebsiella*, *Enterobacter*, *Proteus*, *Pseudomonas*, streptococci, staphylococci
- Nonbacterial prostatitis — unknown

Pathophysiologic changes

Inflammatory response in the prostate ➤	Prostate becoming large, tender, and firm; chills
Blocked urethra by enlarged prostate ➤	Dysuria, nocturia, urinary obstruction
UTI ➤	Cloudy urine, frequent and urgent urination, suprapubic tenderness, dysuria, nocturia
Compression of the prostate gland ➤	Low back pain; perineal fullness
Systemic infection ➤	Fever, myalgia, fatigue, arthralgia

PROSTATIC INFLAMMATION

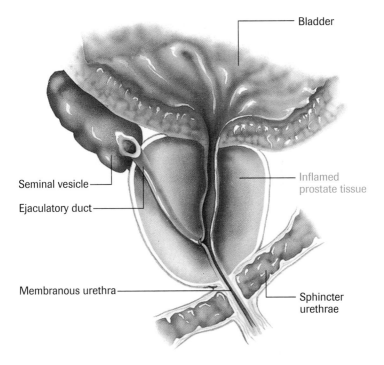

Bladder

Seminal vesicle

Ejaculatory duct

Membranous urethra

Inflamed prostate tissue

Sphincter urethrae

Syphilis

- Contagious, systemic venereal or congenital disease caused by a spirochete
- Begins in the mucous membranes and quickly spreads to nearby lymph nodes and bloodstream
- Transmitted primarily through sexual contact; transmission also possible from mother to fetus

Causes
- *Treponema pallidum*

Pathophysiologic changes

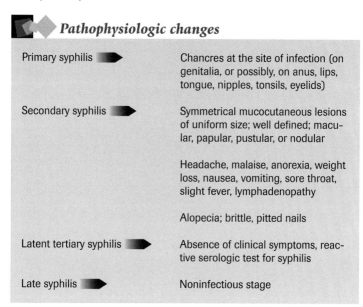

Primary syphilis ➤	Chancres at the site of infection (on genitalia, or possibly, on anus, lips, tongue, nipples, tonsils, eyelids)
Secondary syphilis ➤	Symmetrical mucocutaneous lesions of uniform size; well defined; macular, papular, pustular, or nodular
	Headache, malaise, anorexia, weight loss, nausea, vomiting, sore throat, slight fever, lymphadenopathy
	Alopecia; brittle, pitted nails
Latent tertiary syphilis ➤	Absence of clinical symptoms, reactive serologic test for syphilis
Late syphilis ➤	Noninfectious stage

MANIFESTATIONS OF SYPHILIS

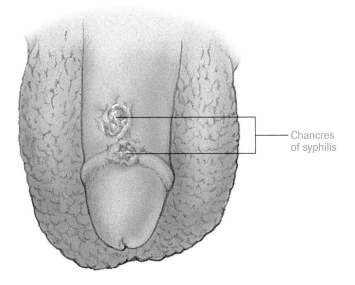

Chancres
of syphilis

Testicular cancer

- Commonly originates in gonadal cells
- About 40% seminomas — uniform, undifferentiated cell resembling primitive gonadal cells; remaining tumors are nonseminomas — tumors showing various degrees of differentiation
- Prognosis dependent on cell type and disease stage; when treated with surgery and radiation, almost all patients with localized disease survive beyond 5 years

Causes
- Unknown

Pathophysiologic changes

Tumor growth ➡	Firm, painless, smooth testicular mass; occasional complaints of heaviness
Tumor production of chorionic gonadotropin or estrogen ➡	Gynecomastia, nipple tenderness
Ureteral obstruction ➡	Urinary complaints
Invasion of the respiratory system ➡	Cough, hemoptysis, shortness of breath
Continued cellular proliferation ➡	Fatigue, anorexia, pallor, lethargy, weight loss

TESTICULAR CANCER

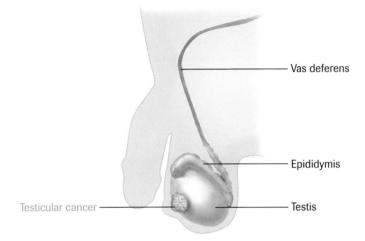

Vas deferens

Epididymis

Testicular cancer

Testis

STAGING TESTICULAR CANCER

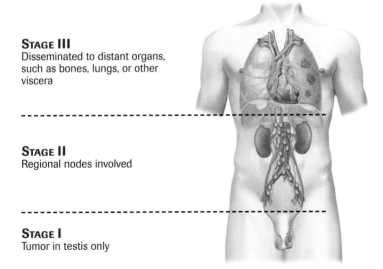

STAGE III
Disseminated to distant organs, such as bones, lungs, or other viscera

STAGE II
Regional nodes involved

STAGE I
Tumor in testis only

Testicular torsion

- Abnormal twisting of the spermatic cord due to rotation of a testis or the mesorchium
- May occur inside or outside the tunica vaginalis
- Intravaginal torsion most common in adolescence; extravaginal, in neonates
- Outcomes ranging from strangulation to eventual infarction of the testis without treatment

Causes
- Extravaginal torsion
  - Loose attachment of the tunica vaginalis to the scrotal lining causing spermatic cord rotation above the testis
  - Sudden forceful contraction of the cremaster muscle due to physical exertion or irritation of the muscle
- Intravaginal torsion
  - Abnormality of coverings of the testis and abnormally positioned testis
  - Incomplete attachment of testis and spermatic fascia to the scrotal wall, leaving testis free to rotate around its vascular pedicle

Pathophysiologic changes

Twisting of arteries and veins in spermatic cord ➡	Excruciating pain in affected testis or iliac fossa of the pelvis; edematous, elevated and ecchymotic scrotum with loss of the cremasteric reflex; vascular engorgement and ischemia; without treatment testis becoming dysfunctional and necrotic

TESTICULAR TORSION

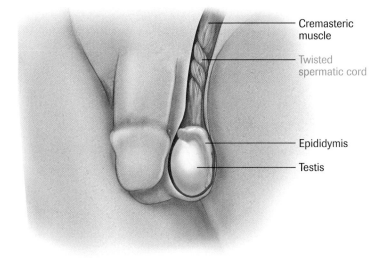

Cremasteric muscle

Twisted spermatic cord

Epididymis

Testis

Trichomoniasis

- Protozoal infection affecting about 15% of sexually active females and 10% of sexually active males
- Common sites of infection in females: vagina, urethra and, possibly, the endocervix, bladder, Bartholin's glands, or Skene's glands; in males: lower urethra and, possibly, the prostate gland, seminal vesicles, or epididymis

Causes
- *Trichomonas vaginalis,* a tetraflagellated, motile protozoa

Pathophysiologic changes

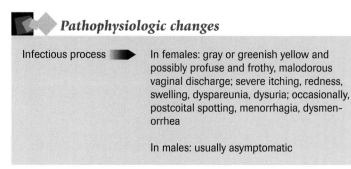

Infectious process ➤ In females: gray or greenish yellow and possibly profuse and frothy, malodorous vaginal discharge; severe itching, redness, swelling, dyspareunia, dysuria; occasionally, postcoital spotting, menorrhagia, dysmenorrhea

In males: usually asymptomatic

MANIFESTATIONS OF TRICHOMONIASIS

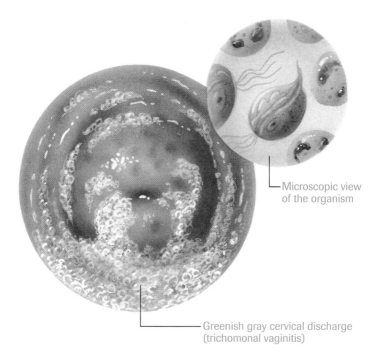

Microscopic view
of the organism

Greenish gray cervical discharge
(trichomonal vaginitis)

Varicocele

- Mass of dilated and tortuous varicose veins in the spermatic cord; commonly described as a "bag of worms"
- Occurs in 30% of men diagnosed with infertility
- More common in men ages 15 to 25

Causes

- Incompetent or congenitally absent valves in spermatic veins
- Tumor or thrombus obstructing the inferior vena cava (unilateral left-sided varicocele)

Pathophysiologic changes

Elevated temperature caused by increased blood flow to the testes ➡	Testicular atrophy, spermatogenesis, and infertility
Pooling of blood ➡	Feeling of heaviness on affected side, testicular pain, and tenderness on palpation

VARICOCELE

Dilated and tortuous veins

Epididymis

Testis

Scrotal sac

Vulvar cancer

- Accounts for approximately 4% of all gynecologic malignancies
- Squamous cell carcinoma most common
- Chance of effective treatment and survival increased by early diagnosis
- If no positive nodes revealed in lymph node dissection, 90% 5-year survival rate; otherwise, 50% to 60%
- May occur at any age, even in infants, but peak incidence after age 60

Causes
- Unknown

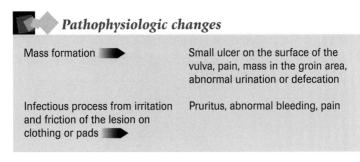

Pathophysiologic changes

Mass formation ➤	Small ulcer on the surface of the vulva, pain, mass in the groin area, abnormal urination or defecation
Infectious process from irritation and friction of the lesion on clothing or pads ➤	Pruritus, abnormal bleeding, pain

CARCINOMA OF THE VULVA

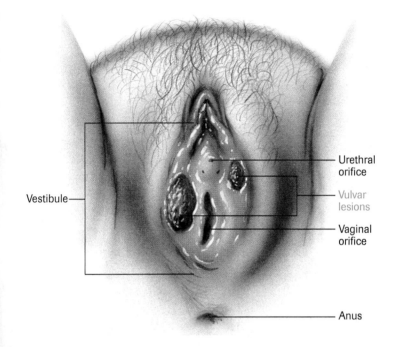

Urethral
orifice

Vulvar
lesions

Vestibule

Vaginal
orifice

Anus

12

Genetic disorders

Cystic fibrosis

- Chronic, progressive dysfunction of exocrine glands affecting multiple organ systems
- Most common fatal genetic disease in white children
- Characterized by chronic airway infection leading to bronchiectasis, bronchiolectasis, exocrine pancreatic insufficiency, intestinal and reproductive dysfunction, and abnormal sweat gland function

Causes

- Genetic mutation on chromosome 7q; transmitted by autosomal recessive inheritance

Pathophysiologic changes

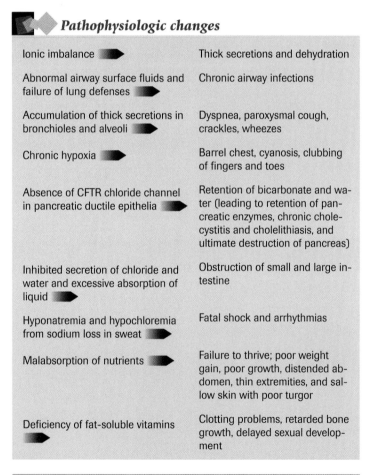

Ionic imbalance	Thick secretions and dehydration
Abnormal airway surface fluids and failure of lung defenses	Chronic airway infections
Accumulation of thick secretions in bronchioles and alveoli	Dyspnea, paroxysmal cough, crackles, wheezes
Chronic hypoxia	Barrel chest, cyanosis, clubbing of fingers and toes
Absence of CFTR chloride channel in pancreatic ductile epithelia	Retention of bicarbonate and water (leading to retention of pancreatic enzymes, chronic cholecystitis and cholelithiasis, and ultimate destruction of pancreas)
Inhibited secretion of chloride and water and excessive absorption of liquid	Obstruction of small and large intestine
Hyponatremia and hypochloremia from sodium loss in sweat	Fatal shock and arrhythmias
Malabsorption of nutrients	Failure to thrive; poor weight gain, poor growth, distended abdomen, thin extremities, and sallow skin with poor turgor
Deficiency of fat-soluble vitamins	Clotting problems, retarded bone growth, delayed sexual development

SYSTEMIC CHANGES IN CYSTIC FIBROSIS

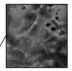

LUNG
Lung tissue shows extensive destruction from obstruction and infection in cystic fibrosis

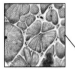

LIVER
Small bile ducts become obstructed and impede digestion

PANCREAS
Ductal occlusion prevents digestive enzymes from being available for digestion

SMALL INTESTINE
Thick stool may obstruct the intestines

REPRODUCTIVE TRACT
About 95% of males are infertile due to the absence of mature sperm; females may be infertile because of a mucus plug that impedes sperm transport into the uterus

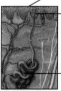

Pore of sweat gland

Eccrine sweat gland

SKIN
Malfunctioning sweat glands secrete sodium chloride

Down syndrome

- Spontaneous chromosome abnormality causing characteristic facial features and other distinctive physical abnormalities (apparent at birth) and mental retardation
- Also called *trisomy 21*
- Carries significantly increased life expectancy due to improved treatment for heart defects, respiratory and other infections, and acute leukemia

Causes

- Chromosomal aberration (three copies of chromosome 21)

Pathophysiologic changes

Chromosomal aberration ➡	Distinct craniofacial features apparent at birth: low nasal bridge, epicanthal folds, protruding tongue, low-set ears, small open mouth and disproportionately large tongue, single transverse crease on palm (simian crease), small white spots on iris (Brushfield's spots), lethargy, mental retardation
Congenital defects ➡	Heart defects, duodenal atresia, Hirschsprung's disease, polydactyly, syndactyly
Hypotonia and decreased cognitive processing ➡	Developmental delay
Decreased muscle tone in limbs ➡	Impaired reflexes

CLINICAL FEATURES OF DOWN SYNDROME

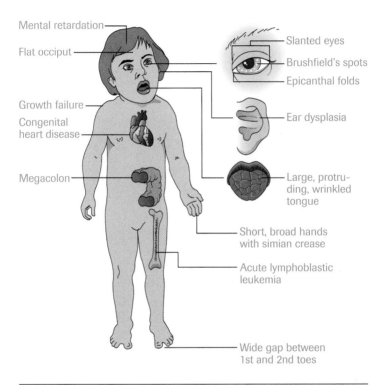

Mental retardation

Flat occiput

Growth failure

Congenital heart disease

Megacolon

Slanted eyes

Brushfield's spots

Epicanthal folds

Ear dysplasia

Large, protruding, wrinkled tongue

Short, broad hands with simian crease

Acute lymphoblastic leukemia

Wide gap between 1st and 2nd toes

Image from Rubin, E., and Farber, J.L. *Pathology,* 3rd ed. Philadelphia: Lippincott Williams & Wilkins, 1999.

Sickle cell anemia

- Congenital hemolytic anemia resulting from defective hemoglobin (Hb) molecules (Hb S); producing characteristic sickle-shaped red blood cells (RBCs)
- Occurs primarily in those of African and Mediterranean descent
- Typically not symptomatic until after age 6 months due to presence of large amount of fetal Hb

Causes

- Autosomal recessive inheritance (homozygous inheritance of Hb S-producing gene)

Pathophysiologic changes

Repeated cycles of deoxygenation and sickling ➤	Anemia, tachycardia, cardiomegaly, chronic fatigue, unexplained dyspnea, hepatomegaly, joint swelling, aching bones
Blood vessel obstruction by rigid, tangled, sickled cells (leading to tissue anoxia and possibly necrosis) ➤	Severe pain in abdomen, thorax, muscles, joints, or bones (characterizes painful crisis); pale lips, tongue, palms, or nail beds; lethargy; listlessness; sleepiness; irritability; severe pain; and fever
Increased bilirubin production ➤	Jaundice, dark urine
Autosplenectomy (splenic damage and scarring occurring with long-term disease) ➤	Aplastic (megaloblastic) crisis: pallor, lethargy, sleepiness, dyspnea, possible coma, markedly decreased bone marrow activity, and RBC hemolysis
Sudden massive entrapment of cells in spleen and liver ➤	Lethargy, pallor, and hypovolemic shock

SICKLE CELL CRISIS

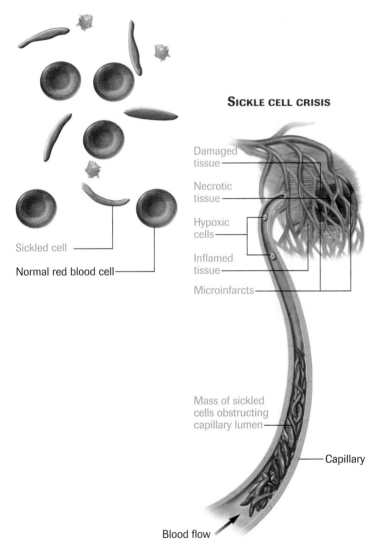

Peripheral Blood Smear in Sickle Cell Anemia

Sickled cell

Normal red blood cell

Sickle Cell Crisis

Damaged tissue

Necrotic tissue

Hypoxic cells

Inflamed tissue

Microinfarcts

Mass of sickled cells obstructing capillary lumen

Capillary

Blood flow

Disorders of electrolyte balance

Electrolyte imbalance	Signs and symptoms
Hyponatremia ▦ Serum sodium < 135 mEq/L (SI, 135 mmol/L)	▦ Muscle twitching and weakness ▦ Lethargy, confusion, seizures, and coma ▦ Hypotension and tachycardia ▦ Nausea, vomiting, and abdominal cramps ▦ Oliguria or anuria
Hypernatremia ▦ Serum sodium > 145 mEq/L (SI, 145 mmol/L)	▦ Agitation, restlessness, fever, and decreased level of consciousness ▦ Muscle irritability and seizures ▦ Hypertension, tachycardia, pitting edema, and excessive weight gain ▦ Thirst, increased viscosity of saliva, and rough tongue ▦ Dyspnea, respiratory arrest, and death
Hypokalemia ▦ Serum potassium < 3.5 mEq/L (SI, 3.5 mmol/L)	▦ Dizziness, hypotension, arrhythmias, electrocardiogram (ECG) changes, and cardiac and respiratory arrest ▦ Nausea, vomiting, anorexia, diarrhea, decreased peristalsis, abdominal distention, and paralytic ileus ▦ Muscle weakness, fatigue, and leg cramps
Hyperkalemia ▦ Serum potassium > 5 mEq/L (SI, 5 mmol/L)	▦ Tachycardia changing to bradycardia, ECG changes, and cardiac arrest ▦ Nausea, diarrhea, and abdominal cramps ▦ Muscle weakness and flaccid paralysis
Hypochloremia ▦ Serum chloride < 100 mEq/L (SI, 100 mmol/L)	▦ Muscle hyperexcitability and tetany ▦ Shallow, depressed breathing ▦ Usually associated with hyponatremia and its characteristic symptoms, such as muscle weakness and twitching
Hyperchloremia ▦ Serum chloride > 108 mEq/L (SI, 108 mmol/L)	▦ Deep, rapid breathing ▦ Weakness ▦ Lethargy, possibly leading to coma
Hypocalcemia ▦ Serum calcium < 8.2 mg/dl (SI, 2.05 mmol/L)	▦ Anxiety, irritability, twitching around the mouth, laryngospasm, seizures, positive Chvostek's and Trousseau's signs ▦ Hypotension and arrhythmias due to decreased calcium influx

Electrolyte imbalance   Signs and symptoms

Electrolyte imbalance	Signs and symptoms
Hypercalcemia ▪ Serum calcium > 10.2 mg/dl (SI, 2.54 mmol/L)	▪ Drowsiness, lethargy, headaches, irritability, confusion, depression, apathy, tingling and numbness of fingers, muscle cramps, and seizures ▪ Weakness and muscle flaccidity ▪ Bone pain and pathological fractures ▪ Heart block ▪ Anorexia, nausea, vomiting, constipation, dehydration, and abdominal cramps ▪ Flank pain
Hypomagnesemia ▪ Serum magnesium < 1.3 mEq/L (SI, 0.65 mmol/L)	▪ Nearly always coexists with hypokalemia and hypocalcemia ▪ Hyperirritability, tetany, leg and foot cramps, positive Chvostek's and Trousseau's signs, confusion, delusions, and seizures ▪ Arrhythmias, vasodilation, and hypotension
Hypermagnesemia ▪ Serum magnesium > 2.1 mEq/dl (SI, 1.05 mmol/L)	▪ Central nervous system depression, lethargy, and drowsiness ▪ Diminished reflexes; muscle weakness to flaccid paralysis ▪ Respiratory depression ▪ Heart block, bradycardia, widened QRS, and prolonged QT interval ▪ Hypotension
Hypophosphatemia ▪ Serum phosphate < 2.7 mg/dl (SI, 0.87 mmol/L)	▪ Muscle weakness, tremor, and paresthesia ▪ Tissue hypoxia ▪ Bone pain, decreased reflexes, and seizures ▪ Weak pulse ▪ Hyperventilation ▪ Dysphagia and anorexia
Hyperphosphatemia ▪ Serum phosphate > 4.5 mg/dl (SI, 1.45 mmol/L)	▪ Usually asymptomatic unless leading to hypocalcemia, then evidenced by tetany and seizures ▪ Hyperreflexia, flaccid paralysis, and muscular weakness

Infectious disorders

Disorder	Characteristics

Bacterial infections

Anthrax

Bacterial infection characterized as cutaneous, inhalational, or intestinal.
- Cutaneous anthrax is characterized by a small, elevated, itchy lesion, which develops into a vesicle and then a painless ulcer, along with enlarged lymph glands.
- Inhalational anthrax is characterized by flulike symptoms, followed by severe respiratory difficulty and shock.
- With intestinal anthrax, fever, nausea, vomiting, and decreased appetite occur, which progress to abdominal pain, hematemesis, and severe diarrhea.

Chlamydia

Sexually transmitted infection caused by *Chlamydia trachomatis.*
- Disease pattern depends on the individual infected and the site of infection.

Conjunctivitis

Bacterial or viral infection of the conjunctiva of the eye.
- Associated with hyperemia of the eye, discharge, tearing, pain, and photophobia.

Gonorrhea

Sexually transmitted infection caused by *Neisseria gonorrhoeae,* a gram-negative, oxidase-positive diplococcus.
- Disease pattern depends on the individual infected and the site of infection.

Listeriosis

Infection caused by weakly hemolytic, gram-positive bacillus *Listeria monocytogenes.*
- Disease may cause abortion, premature delivery, stillbirth, or organ abscesses in fetuses. Neonates may have tense fontanels due to meningitis, be irritabile or lethargic, have seizures, or be comatose.

Lyme disease

Infection caused by spirochets *Borrelia burgdorferi* and transmitted by ixodid tick.
- Typically, causes a ringlike rash, called *erythema chronicum migrans* and may disseminate to other skin sites or organs through the bloodstream or lymphatic system.

Meningitis

Meningeal inflammation caused by bacteria, viruses, protozoa, or fungi.
- Characteristic signs include fever, chills, headache, nuchal rigidity, vomiting, photophobia, lethargy, coma, positive Brudzinki's and Kernig's signs, increased deep tendon reflexes, widened pulse pressure, bradycardia, and rash.

Otitis media

Inflammation of the middle ear caused by a bacterial infection.
- Viral symptoms occur, generally followed by ear pain.

Disorder   Characteristics

Bacterial infections (continued)

Peritonitis | Acute or chronic inflammation of the peritoneum caused by bacterial invasion.
- Onset commonly sudden, with severe and diffuse abdominal pain.

Pertussis (whooping cough) | Highly contagious respiratory infection usually caused by the nonmotile, gram-negative coccobacillus *Bordetella pertussis* and, occasionally, by the related similar bacteria *B. parapertussis* or *B. bronchiseptica*.
- Known for its associated spasmodic cough, characteristically ending in a loud, crowing inspiratory whoop. Complications include apnea, hypoxia, seizures, pneumonia, encephalopathy, and death.

Pneumonia | Infection of the lung parenchyma that's bacterial, fungal, or protozoal in origin.
- Bacterial infection initially triggers alveolar inflammation and edema, which produces an area of low ventilation with normal perfusion. Capillaries become engorged with blood, causing stasis. As alveolocapillary membranes break down, alveoli fill with blood and exudates, causing atelectasis, or lung collapse.

Salmonellosis | Disease caused by a serotype of the genus *Salmonella,* a member of the *Enterobacteriaceae* family.
- Characteristic symptoms include fever, abdominal pain or cramps, and severe diarrhea with enterocolitis.

Shigellosis | Acute intestinal infection caused by the bacteria shigella, a member of the *Enterobacteriaceae* family. It's a short, nonmotile, gram-negative rod.
- Shigella organisms invade the intestinal mucosa and cause inflammation. Symptoms can range from watery stools to fever, cramps, and stools with pus, mucus, or blood.

Tetanus | Acute exotoxin-mediated infection caused by the anaerobic, spore-forming, gram-positive bacillus *Clostridium tetani.*
- Characterized by marked muscle hypertonicity, hyperactive deep tendon reflexes, and painful, involuntary muscle contractions. Severe muscle spasms can last up to 7 days.

Toxic shock syndrome (TSS) | Acute bacterial infection caused by toxin-producing, penicillin-resistant strains of *Staphylococcus aureus,* such as TSS toxin-1 or staphylococcal enterotoxins B and C. It can also be caused by *Streptococcus pyogenes.*
- Signs and symptoms include fever, hypotension, renal failure, and multisystem involvement.

Disorder   Characteristics

Bacterial infections (continued)

Tuberculosis	Infectious disease transmitted by inhaling *Mycobacterium tuberculosis*, an acid-fast bacillus, from an infected person. ■ Characterized by fever, weakness, anorexia, night sweats, weight loss, and cough.
Urinary tract infection	Infection most commonly caused by enteric gram-negative bacilli resulting from microorganisms entering the urethra and then ascending into the bladder. ■ Commonly causes urgency, frequency, and dysuria.

Viral infections

Avian influenza	An influenza A virus that typically infects birds. ■ Reported symptoms in humans include fever, cough, sore throat, and muscle aches and can progress to eye infections, pneumonia, and acute respiratory distress.
Cytomegalovirus infection	A deoxyribonucleic acid (DNA) virus that's a member of the herpes virus group. ■ The virus spreads through the body in lymphocytes or mononuclear cells to the lungs, liver, GI tract, eyes, and central nervous system (CNS), where it commonly produces inflammatory reactions.
Herpes simplex virus (HSV)	HSV is an enveloped, double-stranded DNA virus that causes both herpes simplex type 1 and type 2. Type 1 HSV is transmitted via oral and respiratory secretions; type 2 HSV is transmitted via sexual contact. ■ Characteristic painful, vesicular lesions are usually observed at the site of initial infection.
Herpes zoster	Caused by a reactivation of varicella-zoster virus that has been lying dormant in the cerebral ganglia or the ganglia of posterior nerve roots. ■ Small, painful, red, nodular skin lesions develop on areas along nerve paths and change to vesicles filled with pus or fluid.
Human immunodeficiency virus (HIV) infection	A ribonucleic acid (RNA) retrovirus that causes acquired immunodeficiency deficiency syndrome (AIDS). ■ May remain asymptomatic for years or develop flulike symptoms.
Infectious mononucleosis	Viral illness caused by the Epstein-Barr virus, a B-lymphotropic herpes virus. ■ Dying B cells release the virus into the blood, causing fever, sore throat, fatigue, and cervical lymphadenopathy.

Viral infections (continued)

Disorder	Characteristics
Monkeypox	Rare disease caused by the monkeypox virus, which belongs to the orthopoxvirus group. ▦ In humans, monkeypox causes swollen lymph nodes, fever, headache, muscle aches, backache, exhaustion, and a papular rash with lesions that eventually crust and fall off.
Mumps	Acute viral disease caused by an RNA virus classified as *Rubulavirus* in the *Paramyxoviridae* family. ▦ Characterized by enlargement and tenderness of parotid gland and swelling of other salivary glands.
Rabies	Rapidly progressive infection of the CNS caused by an RNA virus in the *Rhabdoviridae* family transmitted by the bite of an infected animal. ▦ The virus spreads along the nerve pathways to the spinal cord and brain, where it replicates again and causes fever, malaise, headache, anorexia, nauea, and deteriorating neurologic function.
Respiratory syncytial virus	Infection of the respiratory tract caused by an enveloped RNA paramyxovirus. ▦ Bronchiolitis or pneumonia ensues and, in severe cases, may damage the bronchiolar epithelium leading to interalveolar thickening and filling of alveolar spaces with fluid may occur.
Rubella	An enveloped positive-stranded RNA virus classified as a rubivirus in the *Togaviridae* family. ▦ Characteristic maculopapular rash usually begins on the face and then spreads rapidly.
Rubeola	Acute, highly contagious paramyxovirus infection that's spread by direct contact or by contaminated airborne respiratory droplets. ▦ Characterized by Koplik's spots, a pruritic macular rash that becomes papular and erythematous.
Smallpox	Acute contagious virus caused by the variola virus, a member of the *Orthopoxvirus* family. ▦ Sudden onset of influenza-like symptoms including fever, malaise, headache, and severe back pain and a characteristic rash, first on the face, hands, and forearms and then after a few days progressing to the trunk. Lesions also develop in the mucous membranes of the nose and mouth, then ulcerate and release large amounts of virus into the mouth and throat.

Disorder   Characteristics

Viral infections *(continued)*

Varicella (chickenpox)	Common, highly contagious exanthem caused by the varicella-zoster virus, a member of the herpes virus family. ▪ Transmitted by respiratory droplets or contact with vesicles. In utero infection is also possible. ▪ Characterized by a pruritic rash of small, erythematous macules that progresses to papules and then to clear vesicles on an erythematous base.
Viral pneumonia	Lung infection caused by any one of a variety of viruses, transmitted through contact with an infected individual. ▪ Virus invades bronchial mucous glands and goblet cells and leads to fever, rash, diarrhea, and intestinal intussuception.

Fungal infection

Histoplasmosis	Fungal infection caused by *Histoplasma capsulatum,* a dimorphic fungus. ▪ Initially, infected person may be asymptomatic or have symptoms of mild respiratory illness, progressing into more severe illness affecting several organ systems.

Protozoal infections

Toxoplasmosis	Infection caused by the intracellular parasite *Toxoplasma gondii*, which affects both birds and mammals. ▪ Characteristics inlude fever, myalgia, headache, vomiting, neurological changes, and organ failure.
Trichinosis	Infection caused by the parasite *Trichinella spiralis* and transmitted through ingestion of uncooked or undercooked meat that contains encysted larvae. ▪ Characterized by fever, muscle pain, skin lesions, delerium, lethargy, and severe cardiopulmonary or nervous system infections.

Selected references

Albano, C., et al. "Innovations in the Management of Cerebral Injury," *Critical Care Nursing Quarterly* 28(2):135-49, April-June 2005.

Atlas of Pathophysiology, 2nd ed. Philadelphia: Lippincott Williams & Wilkins, 2005.

Breiterman-White, R. "Functional Ability of Patients on Dialysis: The Critical Role of Anemia," *Nephrology Nursing Journal* 32(1):79-82, January-February 2005.

Bridges, E.J., and Dukes, S. "Cardiovascular Aspects of Septic Shock: Pathophysiology, Monitoring, and Treatment," *Critical Care Nurse* 25(2):14-16, 18-20, 22-24, April 2005.

Bristow, N. "Understanding the Symptoms of Irritable Bowel Syndrome," *Nursing Times* 101(10):36-38, March 2005.

Burrows-Hudson, S. "Chronic Kidney Disease: An Overview," *AJN* 105(2):40-49, February 2005.

Deaton, C., and Namasivayam, S. "Nursing Outcomes in Coronary Heart Disease," *Journal of Cardiovascular Nursing* 19(5):308-15, September-October 2004.

Elgart, H.N. "Assessment of Fluids and Electrolytes," *ACCN Clinical Issues* 15(4):607-21, October-December 2004.

Farquhar, S.L., and Fantasia, L. "Pulmonary Anatomy and Physiology of the Effects of COPD," *Home Healthcare Nurse* 23(3):167-66, March 2005.

Giger, J.N. "Understanding Genetics: The Relationship of Disease and Genetic Predisposition in African-Americans," *Journal of National Black Nurses' Association* 15(2):vii-viii, December 2004.

Just the Facts: Pathophysiology. Philadelphia: Lippincott Williams & Wilkins, 2005.

Lomborg, K., et al. "Body Care Experienced by People Hospitalized with Severe Respiratory Disease," *Journal of Advanced Nursing* 50(3):262-71, May 2005.

Maxwell, C., and Viale, P.H. "Cancer Treatment-Induced Bone Loss in Patients with Breast or Prostate Cancer," *Oncology Nursing Forum* 32(3):589-603, May 2005.

Nicholson, C. "Cardiovascular Care of Patients with Marfan Syndrome," *Nursing Standard* 19(27):38-44, March 2005.

Professional Guide to Pathophysiology. Philadelphia: Lippincott Williams & Wilkins, 2003.

Pruitt, B., and Jacobs, M. "Caring for a Patient with Asthma," *Nursing* 35(2):48-51, February 2005.

Ryan, C.J., and Zerwic, J.J. "Knowledge of Symptom Clusters Among Adults at Risk for Acute Myocardial Infarction," *Nursing Research* 53(6):363-69, November-December 2004.

Sheerin, F. "Spinal Cord Injury: Anatomy and Physiology of the Spinal Cord," *Emergency Nurse* 12(8):30-36, December 2004.

Smeltzer, S.C., and Bare, B.G. *Brunner and Suddarth's Textbook of Medical-Surgical Nursing*, 10th ed. Philadelphia: Lippincott Williams & Wilkins, 2004.

Thompson, C., and Tsiperfal, A. "Is There an Output Failure?" *Progress in Cardiovascular Nursing* 20(2):98, Spring 2005.

Index

i refers to an illustration; t refers to a table.

i refers to an illustration; t refers to a table.

C

---

i refers to an illustration; t refers to a table.

---

i refers to an illustration; t refers to a table.

i refers to an illustration; t refers to a table.

Gout, 228
  of foot, 229i
  of knee, 229i
Graves' disease, histologic changes in, 303i
Guillain-Barré syndrome, 126
  peripheral nerve demyelination in, 127i

H

Hashimoto's thyroiditis, histologic changes in, 305i
Hearing loss, 128
  conductive, causes of, 129i
Heart failure, 28
  left-sided, 28, 29i
  right-sided, 28, 29i
Hematologic system, 248-275
Hemophilia, 264
  clotting in, 265i
Hemorrhoids, 188, 189i
Hepatitis, viral, 190
  liver biopsy results in, 191i
Hernia
  hiatal, 192, 193i
  inguinal, 196, 197i
Herniated intervertebral disk, 130
  pain pathway in, 131i
Herpes simplex type 2, 382, 383i
Herpes simplex virus, 424t
Herpes zoster, 352, 353i, 424t
Hiatal hernia, 192, 193i
Hirschsprung's disease, 194
  bowel dilation in, 195i
Histoplasmosis, 426t
Hives, 364, 365i
Hodgkin's disease, 266
  Ann Arbor staging system for, 267i
Human immunodeficiency virus infection, 278, 424t
  manifestations of, 279i
Hydrocele, 384, 385i
Hydrocephalus, 132
  ventricular enlargement in, 133i
Hydronephrosis, 324
  renal damage in, 325i
Hypercalcemia, 421t

i refers to an illustration; t refers to a table.

i refers to an illustration; t refers to a table.

i refers to an illustration; t refers to a table.

i refers to an illustration; t refers to a table.

i refers to an illustration; t refers to a table.

---

i refers to an illustration; t refers to a table.

Squamous cell carcinoma, 362, 363i
Stomach ulcers, 214, 215i
Strains, 242, 243i
Stroke, 160
    ischemic, 161i
Syndrome of inappropriate antidiuretic hormone, 308, 309i
Syphilis, 398
    manifestations of, 399i
Systemic lupus erythematosus, 290
    effects of, 291i

T

Tendinitis, 244
    in elbow, 245i
Tension pneumothorax, 86, 87i
Testicular cancer, 400, 401i
    staging of, 401i
Testicular torsion, 402, 403i
Tetanus, 423t
Tetralogy of Fallot, 60, 61i
Thalassemia, 274
    peripheral blood smear in, 275i
Thyroid cancer, 310, 311i
Thyroid gland, 303i
Thyroid storm, 302
Thyrotoxicosis. *See* Hyperthyroidism.
Toxic shock syndrome, 423t
Toxoplasmosis, 426t
Transposition of the great arteries, 62, 63i
Trichinosis, 426t
Trichomoniasis, 404
    manifestations of, 405i
Tuberculosis, 98, 424t
    appearance of, on lung tissue, 99i

U

Ulcerative colitis, 212
    mucosal changes in, 213i
Ulcers, 214
    types and sites of, 215i
Upper respiratory tract infection, 100
    complications of, 101i
Urinary tract infection, 424t

i refers to an illustration; t refers to a table.

Urticaria, 364, 365i
Uterine fibroids, 380, 381i

V

Varicella, 426t
Varicocele, 406, 407i
Ventricular septal defect, 64, 65i
Viral infections, 424-426t
Viral pneumonia, 426t
Vulvar cancer, 408, 409i

WXYZ

Warts, 366
    cross section of, 367i
    periungual, 367i
West Nile encephalitis, 162
    cerebral edema in, 163i
Whiplash. *See* Acceleration-deceleration injuries.
Whooping cough, 423t

i refers to an illustration; t refers to a table.